Journey from Cognition to Brain to Gene

D0795590

AUG 2 2 2002

WITHDRAWN

FEB 2 4 2023

DAVID O. MCKAY LIBRARY
BYU-IDAHO

PROPER
DAVID O. MCKAY LIBRARY
BYU-IDAHO
REXBURG ID 83460-0405

Journey from Cognition to Brain to Gene

Perspectives from Williams Syndrome

Edited by Ursula Bellugi and Marie St. George

with contributions from
Albert M. Galaburda
Julie R. Korenberg
Debra L. Mills
Allan L. Reiss

A Bradford Book

The MIT Press
Cambridge, Massachusetts
London, England

© 2001 Massachusetts Institute of Technology

All rights reserved. No part of this book may be reproduced in any form by any electronic or mechanical means (including photocopying, recording, or information storage and retrieval) without permission in writing from the publisher.

This book was set in Times New Roman by Graphic Composition, Inc. in QuarkXPress.

Printed and bound in the United States of America.

Library of Congress Cataloging-in-Publication Data

Journey from cognition to brain to gene : perspectives from Williams Syndrome / edited by Ursula Bellugi and Marie St. George ; with contributions from Albert Galaburda . . . [et al.].
    p. ; cm.
  "A Bradford book."
  Includes bibliographical references and index.
  ISBN 0-262-52312-4 (pbk. : alk. paper)
    1. Williams syndrome—Pathophysiology.   2. Williams syndrome—Genetic aspects.
  3. Cognition disorders in children.   I. Bellugi, Ursula, 1931–   II. St. George, Marie.
  III. Galaburda, Albert M., 1948–
    [DNLM: 1. Williams Syndrome—genetics.   2. Brain—pathology.   3. Cognition—physiology.
  4. Williams Syndrome—physiopathology.   5. Williams Syndrome—psychology. QS 677 J86 2001]
  RJ506.W44 J68 2001
  618.92′0042—dc21

                                                                                    00-054892

We dedicate this book to the families and individuals with Williams Syndrome who have contributed so much of their time and effort cheerfully and willingly to take part in the research represented in this book. We have worked closely with the Williams Syndrome Association, an organization devoted to improving the lives of individuals with Williams Syndrome and their families, since its early days in 1984. As a gesture of our gratitude to the individuals and their families, the proceeds from this book will be directed to the Williams Syndrome Association.

Contents

On the Cover: A composite of images taken from the integrated studies represented in this book. The centerpiece is a picture of a child with Williams Syndrome, surrounded by images of: 1) language and spatial abilities (Bellugi); 2) brain structure (Reiss); 3) a neurophysiological marker (Mills); 4) the molecular genetic structure of Williams Syndrome (Korenberg).

Contributors

Ralph Adolphs
Department of Neurology
University of Iowa Hospitals and Clinics
Iowa City, Iowa

Twyla D. Alvarez
Department of Neurosciences
University of California at San Diego
La Jolla, California

Lawrence G. Appelbaum
Center for Research in Language
University of California, San Diego
La Jolla, California

Ursula Bellugi
Laboratory for Cognitive Neuroscience
The Salk Institute for Biological Studies
La Jolla, California

Dennis Burian
Department of Chemistry and
Biochemistry
University of Oklahoma
Norman, Oklahoma

Xiao-Ning Chen
Medical Genetics
Cedars-Sinai Medical Center
Los Angeles, California

Michael Chiles
Laboratory for Cognitive Neuroscience
The Salk Institute for Biological Studies
La Jolla, California

Stephan Eliez
Department of Psychiatry and
Behavioral Sciences
Stanford University School of Medicine
Stanford, California

Albert M. Galaburda
Department of Neurology
Beth Israel Deaconess Medical Center
and Harvard University Medical School
Boston, Massachusetts

Hamao Hirota
Medical Genetics
Cedars-Sinai Medical Center
Los Angeles, California

Wendy Jones
Laboratory for Cognitive Neuroscience
The Salk Institute for Biological Studies
La Jolla, California

Julie R. Korenberg
Medical Genetics
Cedars-Sinai Medical Center
Los Angeles, California

Zona Lai
Laboratory for Cognitive Neuroscience
The Salk Institute for Biological Studies
La Jolla, California

Liz Lichtenberger
Laboratory for Cognitive Neuroscience
The Salk Institute for Biological Studies
La Jolla, California

Alan Lincoln
Laboratory of Developmental
Neuropsychology
California School of Professional
Psychology
San Diego, California

Rumiko Matsuoka
Pediatric Cardiology
The Heart Institute of Japan
Tokyo, Japan

Debra L. Mills
Center for Research in Language
University of California, San Diego
La Jolla, California

Helen Neville
University of Oregon
Eugene, Oregon

Judy Reilly
Department of Psychology
San Diego State University
San Diego, California

Allan L. Reiss
Department of Psychiatry and
Behavioral Sciences
Stanford University School of Medicine
Stanford, California

Bruce Roe
Department of Chemistry and
Biochemistry
University of Oklahoma
Norman, Oklahoma

Marie St. George
Center for Research in Language
University of California, San Diego
La Jolla, California

J. Eric Schmitt
Department of Psychiatry and
Behavioral Sciences
Stanford University School of Medicine
Stanford, California

Erica Straus
Department of Psychiatry and
Behavioral Sciences
Stanford University School of Medicine
Stanford, California

Preface

Late one evening in 1985 the phone rang in Dr. Ursula Bellugi's lab at the Salk Institute. The woman on the phone began by saying "Noam Chomsky told me to call you . . ." The woman described her daughter, age 14, who seemed to have a rare syndrome in which her engaging language abilities remarkably masked her low IQ of 49. After some coaxing, as this was not her area of expertise, Bellugi reluctantly agreed to meet with the child who had been diagnosed with Williams Syndrome (WMS). In an exciting first meeting, the girl exemplified what would turn out to be one of the hallmarks of the syndrome: a dissociation between visuospatial and language abilities (see Figure 1). Her drawing of an elephant was unrecognizable without the verbal labels we added as she talked her way through the drawing. In contrast, her description of an elephant was grammatically fluent with complex sentences including what an elephant is, what it does, what it has ("It has a long trunk that can pick up grass or pick up hay . . . you don't want an elephant as a pet, you want a cat or a dog or a bird"). Bellugi agreed to meet with the child weekly, and every imaginable cognitive test was given to her over the following year in an attempt to begin to understand what appeared to be an unusual profile of the syndrome in one individual. At the time these studies began, Bellugi had expertise in the effects of right and left hemisphere lesions and the relative sparing and impairment of language and spatial abilities, resulting from her studies of the neurobiology of language in deaf signers. Although not known at the time, this would turn out to be an interesting background with which to approach the WMS puzzle.

Near the end of this initial year of testing, the first meeting of a Williams Syndrome Association was held in San Diego in 1984, with several families attending. At this time there were only 60 identified cases of WMS in the country. Nothing was known of the genetics of the syndrome. In fact little had been published at all on WMS other than a few studies of IQ, which were inconclusive. A medical intern had begun to study the possible contribution of high levels of calcium in the blood to the syndrome. This idea sparked a first attempt at finding the gene associated with WMS based on the hypothesis that it might be related to calcitonin gene related peptide. This first attempt, however, was not as fruitful as the following one would be.

The first big breakthrough came during the next decade, as Bellugi built up a laboratory dedicated in part to the study of the cognitive and brain bases of Williams Syndrome contrasted with Down Syndrome (DNS), with the help of grants from NICHD, NINDS, and NIDCD. She began to uncover the fascinating phenotypic profile of WMS, leading to a series of papers, and a growing interest in Williams Syndrome. A second breakthrough occurred around 1993, when it was discovered that the gene for elastin was part of the microdeletion in WMS (Ewart et al., 1993; Bellugi & Morris, 1995). The road was paved for a molecular genetics branch of the study of WMS. Who would do it? During the whole of her career at The Salk Institute, Bellugi had yearned

Disparate Abilities in One Mind

Elephant Drawing

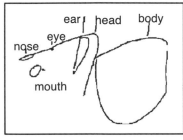

WMS Age 15, IQ 49

Elephant Description

And what an elephant is, it is one of the animals. And what the elephant does, it lives in the jungle. It can also live in the zoo. And what it has, it has long gray ears, fan ears, ears that can blow in the wind. It has a long trunk that can pick up grass, or pick up hay...If they're in a bad mood it can be terrible...If the elephant gets mad it could stomp; it could charge. Sometimes elephants can charge. They have big long tusks. They can damage a car...It could be dangerous. When they're in a pinch, when they're in a bad mood it can be terrible. You don't want an elephant as a pet. You want a cat or a dog or a bird...

Figure 1
The dissociation between language and spatial cognition in WMS is evident in this contrast between the drawing and verbal description of an elephant by a teenager with WMS (Full Scale IQ of 49, Verbal IQ of 52, and Performance IQ of 54).

to be able to integrate results from cognition, brain, and molecular genetics. This was perhaps her chance. After studying WMS individuals for years, developing a cognitive phenotype, uncovering aspects of the brain bases of WMS, setting up a WMS clinic, organizing local, regional and national family meetings, and contributing regularly to the family newsletter, in 1994–1995 Bellugi and colleagues began a program project through NICHD that was one of the first of its kind—to investigate this genetically based syndrome with its well defined phenotype across cognitive, neuroanatomical, neurophysiological, and molecular genetic levels as opposed to merely for the investigation of mental retardation. She gathered a team of scientists whose research is included in this book to participate in the program project. One of the strengths of this book is that all of the levels, from cognition to brain structure, brain function, and molecular genetics, are investigated with the *same* individuals with WMS (with the exception of the cytoarchitectonic studies). The team of scientists have been working together for the same program project focusing on Williams syndrome. See Figure 2 for a diagram of the levels of the program project represented by chapters in this book.

As this book unfolds, you will learn that WMS is a special syndrome for many reasons. As Jonas Salk said of WMS, "I never knew talent was a birth defect." The dis-

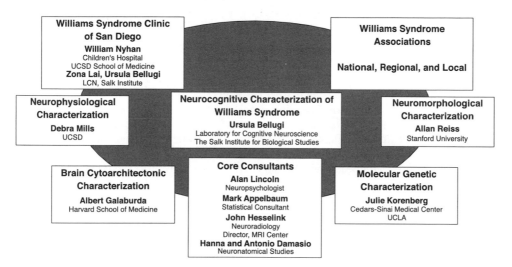

Figure 2
The organization of the Program Project (PPG), from National Institutes of Child Health and Human Development (NICHD PO1 HD 33113). The research in this book stems from studies under this grant involving adolescents and adults with Williams or Down Syndrome. The chart represents the major projects of the program project, each of which is represented in one of the chapters in this issue: Neurocognitive characterization at The Salk Institute (Bellugi et al., chap. 1, and Jones et al., chap. 2); Neurophysiological characterization at UCSD (Mills et al., chap. 3); Neuromorphological characterization at Stanford University (Reiss et al., chap. 4); Brain cytoarchitectonics at Harvard Medical School (Galaburda and Bellugi, chap. 5); and Molecular genetic characterization at Cedars-Sinai Hospital and University of California, Los Angeles (Korenberg et al., chap. 6). The special power of these studies is that the same individuals are carefully screened and diagnosed, and then undergo the same probes across multiple levels and disciplines. Studies of infants and children with Williams and Down Syndrome are supported as part of two center grants from National Institute of Deafness and Other Communication Disorders (DC 02189) and from National Institute of Neurological Diseases and Stroke (NS 22342).

crepancy between language ability and IQ is startling, and many who hear about the syndrome are skeptical until they meet someone with WMS. Their remarkable language provides a window into what it is like to have WMS in that it allows them to be able to explain eloquently what it feels like to be mentally retarded. It is difficult to grasp their sophistication with language, their connection to their own emotions, and their ability to express those emotions without actually talking to someone with WMS. Below is an excerpt from an interview with Bellugi and twins, both men age 32, with WMS. The first quote is from one twin, the second from the other twin, when asked what they would want other people to know about WMS.

It is what you're born with, it is what you have to accept, and it is something that you go on day to day, year to year, month to month with. And no matter how people treat people with Williams Syndrome, you always have to stand tall and ignore the things that are said because they are, they don't understand the things that we go through every day that we wake up. We should be treated the same way somebody else should be treated. Even when times are bad we still try to shine a light upon other people, and to give that sense of glow to our friends . . . You have to accept things you cannot change. (Twin #1).

We are respectable, loving, understanding people. With pride, and dignity, and grace. And people should understand that Williams Syndrome people don't really care about the bad things in life and what goes on in the world because we as people have enough problems of our own living day to day . . . First of all I am a human being, and I'm a man, and I'm an older adult. And I want people to realize that I do have feelings, I'm not a freak . . . So respectability is a main factor in learning how to deal with people with Williams Syndrome or any other syndrome. (Twin #2).

I gotta tell you, Dr. Bellugi, we love everyone that we meet. And if people would be, show us love and kind that we try so much to do to other people, I think doors would open and people would understand that, um, we don't need to carry on wars, that we don't need to carry on gang violence. Peace and love. And that's all that everyone with Williams Syndrome has been asking for years. For someone to give us a break. As much as the break we have been giving to them. (Twin #1).

In addition to expressing themselves linguistically with clarity and eloquence, they frequently take up another form of self-expression, with similarly remarkable performance, in the form of music. People with WMS seem to have a special love of music—both playing instruments and singing, as well as listening to others make music. There are many anecdotes about WMS and music. The fact is that there is something very special about both their attraction as well as their ability to perform. Some can't tie their shoes but can repeat and create complex rhythms on a musical instrument. The incidence of perfect pitch may be greater in WMS than in the general population. Several people with WMS can play a song on the piano after listening to it once. One woman with WMS can sing over a thousand songs in 22 different languages. In one of our first experiences with WMS and music, we discovered a love song written by a woman with WMS to a man with DNS. It was a touching song, to her "sweet petunia."

History of Williams Syndrome

Williams Syndrome was discovered independently by Fanconi (1952) and Williams, a British cardiologist (Williams, Barrett-Boyes, & Lowe, 1961). The name Williams is the one that stuck. Early on, the disorder was also called Williams–Beuran syndrome, as well as Infantile Hypercalcemia. Since 1993, we have learned that WMS is caused by the deletion of one copy of a small set of genes on chromosome 7 (7q11.23), which in-

Photos of Children with Williams Syndrome

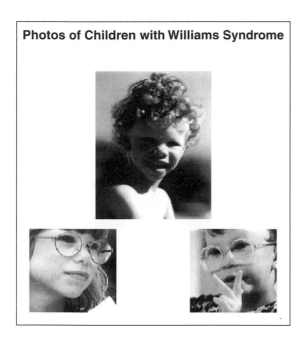

Figure 3
Photos of individuals with Williams Syndrome. Note the similarity in facial features. (Used with permission.)

cludes the genes which code for elastin, LIM1kinase, Frizzled, WSCR1, and Syntaxin1A among others (Korenberg, Chen, Lai et al., 1997; Ewart et al., 1993). The syndrome occurs in approximately 1 in 30,000 births. Some of the frequent physical manifestations of WMS include a specific heart defect (a narrowing of the aorta), a defect in the production of elastin, and hypercalcemia. Their facial features are quite distinctive, and have been described as "pixie-like" and "elfin." People with WMS often look more like each other than they do to people in their own families (see Figure 3 for a collage of photographs). In fact, later in the interview with the WMS twins quoted earlier, they were asked what it felt like to finally meet other people with WMS at a WMS convention. They had never seen anyone else with WMS, other than each other, and at age 30 or so, they met a room full of other WMS people. The first twin said that upon seeing a room full of WMS, he thought, "This is like a giant *cloning convention!*"

Today special schools and music camps for WMS are springing up in many places. Publicity abounds, with stories about Williams Syndrome in the *New York Times, Discover,* and *Newsweek* and on *Nightline, 60 Minutes,* National Public Radio, several PBS and BBC programs including one with Oliver Sacks, as well as articles in the international press. The scientific community has responded with just as much enthusiasm as the popular media. Studying WMS turned out to be a "geneticist's dream," in the words of Julie Korenberg, and progress in this area is advancing at an amazing rate.

An Integrated Program of Research from Cognition to Neural Systems to Genetics

The scientists who are first authors of the chapters in this book represent heads of projects of a large program project from NIH whose ongoing aim is to build bridges across disciplines, linking higher cognitive functions, their underlying neurobiological bases and their molecular genetic underpinnings, using Williams Syndrome as a model (see Figure 2). Williams Syndrome is an ideal model in part because of the principled dissociations among cognitive domains it exhibits. In chapters 1 and 2, Ursula Bellugi and Wendy Jones provide a neurocognitive and social characterization of Williams Syndrome; in chapters 3, 4, and 5, Debra Mills, Allan Reiss, and Albert Galaburda illuminate the neural systems underlying Williams Syndrome using neurophysiological, neuromorphological, and brain cytoarchitectonic approaches, and in Chapter 6, Julie Korenberg probes the depths of the genome structure and aspects of its relation to the cognitive map of Williams Syndrome. The collaboration of these scientists from such diverse levels of science studying the same syndrome is a clear strength of the chapters represented in this book.

Chapter 1, "The Neurocognitive Profile of Williams Syndrome: A Complex Pattern of Strengths and Weaknesses" (Bellugi et al.), introduces dissociations in the cognitive profile of WMS. General cognitive functioning typical of WMS is thoroughly detailed and referenced to normal controls and an age and IQ-matched group with Down Syndrome as well as to several other contrast groups. In addition, the developmental time-course for cognitive domains is illuminated. While there are fascinating peaks in abilities associated with WMS, as we have been discussing, there are also dramatic valleys. Although language processing and face recognition are remarkably "spared," their visuospatial skills are exceedingly poor. The juxtaposition of poor visuospatial skills and near normal face recognition—two visual domains—is explored in this chapter, as well as the intriguing apparent separation between language and general cognitive functioning.

Chapter 2, "Hypersociability: The Social and Affective Phenotype of Williams Syndrome" (Jones et al.), presents a different aspect of the behavioral profile: the dramatic hypersociability in WMS. When coupled with their linguistic abilities, the hypersociability of WMS often keeps people from guessing that they are mentally retarded. They are socially forward and carry on conversations with such ease that it is not until it becomes obvious during the course of conversation that they do not know some fact that most people know—for example, that the sun rises in the east—that you might realize they are mentally retarded. Sociability in WMS was investigated with a number of experiments, testing such things as linguistic affect in storytelling and rating the approachability of unfamiliar faces, as well as data from questionnaires and interviews. Both the experimental and the descriptive data are contrasted with data from normal controls as well as those with DNS and autism. The differences are striking.

Chapter 3, "Neurophysiological Markers of Face Processing in Williams Syndrome" (Mills et al.), examines the organization of brain activity linked to relatively spared cognitive functions in WMS. Using event-related brain potentials (ERPs), they tested the hypothesis that brain systems mediating these seemingly spared cognitive functions, namely, language and face processing, may be abnormally organized in individuals with Williams Syndrome. Specifically, is the organization similar to that of a normal brain at an earlier point in development (which would indicate normal but delayed brain development), or are WMS brains processing information in a different way? In light of previous research on normal developmental changes in the functional organization of the brain, they have identified two domain-specific electrophysiological markers of abnormal brain function in Williams Syndrome. The abnormal morphology in the ERPs for both face processing and for auditory language processing has been observed in virtually all of over 50 adults and children tested with Williams Syndrome. In contrast, these patterns have not been observed in normal adults, children, or infants at any age, nor in any other populations studied. In both language and face processing, the closer the behavioral performance of WMS came to normal, the more unusual their ERP components looked.

In chapter 4, "Neuroanatomy of Williams Syndrome: A High-Resolution MRI Study" (Reiss et al.), neuroimages of individuals with WMS are analyzed and compared with those of normal controls. Overall, those with WMS had decreased brain and cerebral volumes, relative preservation in cerebellar and superior temporal regions, and a substantial decrease in the volume of the brainstem. Additionally, the cerebral gray matter in WMS subjects was relatively preserved compared to controls. However, they had disproportionately low white matter volume. The different cerebral lobe volumes are also reported for both groups, and results are discussed with relation to the molecular genetics, the neurocognitive profile and the neurophysiology of WMS. Hypotheses regarding, for example, what the larger-than-normal gray matter volume of the superior temporal region in WMS might reflect in terms of WMS cognition, are suggested.

Chapter 5, "Cellular and Molecular Cortical Neuroanatomy in Williams Syndrome" (Galaburda & Bellugi), begins to link the anatomical findings to both the genetic as well as the behavioral aspects of the disorder. Galaburda employs an even finer level of analysis of the neuroanatomical data through the use of autopsy specimens. He examined blocks of tissue selected from most classes of cortex from several WMS brains for architectonic differentiation. The WMS brains were studied at four levels: (1) gross anatomy (brain shape, cortical folding, asymmetry), (2) cytoarchitectonic appearance of the cortex, (3) histometric measurements (neuron size and packing density), and (4) immunocytochemistry results. A consistent gross neuroanatomical finding is the abnormal length of the central sulcus, producing an unusual configuration of the dorsal central region, including the dorsal portions of the superior parietal lobe and the dorsal frontal gyrus. The WMS brains also show a lack of asymmetry in the planum temporale, abnormalities in cortical folding, and some curtailment in posterior regions. Most regions show normal cortical cytoarchitecture; however, area 17 shows increased cell size and decreased cell packing density, which suggests the possibility of abnormal connectivity in this region. In an attempt to link genetics to neuroanatomy, molecular observations of Elastin and LIM kinase staining are reported, as both of these proteins are products of the genes that are included in the WMS deletion.

Chapter 6, "Genome Structure and Cognitive Map of Williams Syndrome" (Korenberg et al.), elucidates why the unusual neurocognitive profile of WMS makes it a compelling model of the pathways between genes and human cognition. A unique genomic organization may make WMS an important model of human chromosomal evolution and disease as well. WMS is known to be caused by a small deletion on chromosome 7 that includes the gene encoding elastin (ELN), and up to 20 other genes. The WMS region was analyzed in a large panel of subjects for whom the neurocognitive profile, brain structure and function were also determined. Korenberg et al. describe a model of genome organization, deletion structure, and evolution of the 7q11.2 region. WMS is located within a largely single copy region of chromosome 7 that is flanked by an array of genomic duplications, part of which were duplicated in primate evolution. WMS with typical deletions show no significant evidence of genetic imprinting on neurocognition; however, WMS subjects with smaller deletions suggest candidate regions for parts of the cognitive phenotypic profile. These exciting data may ultimately provide tools for investigating the mechanisms of primate evolution and human cognition.

The contents of this book represent a synthesis of cross-disciplinary research, and provide opportunities to explore some of the central issues of cognitive neuroscience that tie cognitive functions to brain organization and ultimately to the gene.
—La Jolla, California

Ursula Bellugi and Marie St. George are editors of this book. Ursula Bellugi is Professor and Director of the Laboratory for Cognitive Neuroscience at The Salk Institute for Biological Studies. Marie St. George is a scientist with the Center for Research in Language at the University of California, San Diego.

Note

The chapters in this volume appeared in a Special Issue for the *Journal of Cognitive Neuroscience* "Linking Cognitive Neuroscience and Molecular Genetics: New Perspectives from Williams Syndrome" (Volume 12 Supplement, Number 1, 2000). Some changes and updates were made to the chapters between publication in the Special Issue and this volume, and an epilogue was added. Portions of these chapters were originally presented at a Symposium called "Williams Syndrome: Linking Cognition, Brain and Gene," for the Fifth Annual Meeting of the Cognitive Neuroscience Society, in San Francisco in early April 1998. Subsequently, Marie St. George published a review of the meeting and the symposium called "What Studying Genetically Based Disorders Can Tell Us about Ourselves" in *Trends in Cognitive Sciences* (1998), in which she wrote, "One thing that was clear from all of the presenters was that they were excited about the project and the nature of the collaboration." A natural outcome was the proposal to develop these presentations as a Special Issue of the *Journal of Cognitive Neuroscience,* and now a book, with contributions from cognitive neuroscience to molecular genetics.

Acknowledgments

The studies of adolescent and adult Williams, Down, and Normal Controls reported in this book are supported by a Program Project Grant from National Institute of Child Health and Human Development (PO1 HD 33113) to Ursula Bellugi, Program Director. Principal Investigators on the Program Project are authors of chapters in this book (Ursula Bellugi, Neurocognitive Characterization; Debra Mills, Neurophysiological Characterization; Allan Reiss, Neuromorphological Characterization; Albert Galaburda, Brain Cytoarchitectonic Characterization; and Julie R. Korenberg, Molecular Genetic Characterization). Studies of Williams and Down Syndrome individuals in infancy and early childhood, contrasted with individuals with early focal lesions, with language impairment, and with normal controls are supported by National Institute on Deafness and Other Communication Disorders (DC 01289) and National Institute of Neurological Diseases and Stroke (NS 22342) as well as the James S. McDonnell Foundation and the Oak Tree Philanthropic Foundation. We are grateful to individuals with Williams and Down Syndrome and their families who have taken part in these studies, as well as to the Local, National, and Regional Williams Syndrome Associations and Down Syndrome Associations.

References

Bellugi, U. (Symposium Organizer). (April, 1998). Symposium, Bridging cognition, brain and gene: Evidence from Williams syndrome. Cognitive Neuroscience Society Annual Meeting, San Francisco, CA.

Bellugi, U., Lichtenberger, L., Jones, W., Lai, Z., & St. George, M. (chap. 1). The neurocognitive profile of Williams Syndrome: A complex pattern of strengths and weaknesses.

Bellugi, U., & Morris, C. A. (Eds.) (1995). Williams syndrome: From cognition to gene. Abstracts from the Williams Syndrome Association Professional Conference. Special Issue, *Genetic Counseling, 6(1),* 131–192.

Blakeslee, S. (1994). Odd disorder of brain may offer new clues to basis of language. *New York Times,* Science Section, August 2.

Ewart, A., Morris, C., Atkinson, D., Jin, W., Sternes, K., Spallone, P., Stock, A., Leppert, M., & Keating, M. (1993). Hemizygosity at the elastin locus in a developmental disorder, Williams–Beuren syndrome. *Nature Genetics, 5,* 11–16.

Fanconi, G. (1952). In W. R. F. Collis (Ed.), *Textbook of pediatrics* (E. Kawerau, Co-ed. and Trans.). London: Wm. Heinemann.

Galaburda, A., & Bellugi, U. (chap. 5). Cellular and molecular cortical neuroanatomy in Williams Syndrome.

Jones, W., Bellugi, U., Lai, Z., Chiles, M., Reilly, J., Lincoln, A., & Adolphs, R. (chap. 2). Hypersociability: The social and affective phenotype of Williams Syndrome.

Korenberg, J., Chen, X-N., Hirota, H., Lai, Z., Bellugi, U., Burian, D., Roe, B., & Matsuoka, R. (chap. 6). Genome structure and cognitive map of Williams Syndrome.

Korenberg, J. R., Chen, X-N., Lai, Z., Yimlamai, D., Bisighini, R., & Bellugi, U. (1997). Williams Syndrome: The search for the genetic origins of cognition. *American Journal Human Genetics, 61(4),* 103, #579.

Mills, D., Alvarez, T., St. George, M., Appelbaum, L., Bellugi, U., & Neville, H. (chap. 3). Neurophysiological markers of face processing in Williams Syndrome.

Reiss, A., Eliez, S., Schmitt, E., Straus, E., Lai, Z., Jones, W., & Bellugi, U. (chap. 4). Neuroanatomy of Williams Syndrome: A high-resolution MRI study.

St. George, M. (1998). What studying genetically based disorders can tell us about ourselves. *Trends in Cognitive Sciences, 2(6),* 203–204.

Williams, J. C. P., Barratt-Boyes, B. G., & Lowe, J. B. (1961). Supravalvular aortic stenosis. *Circulation, 24,* 1311.

1 The Neurocognitive Profile of Williams Syndrome: A Complex Pattern of Strengths and Weaknesses

Ursula Bellugi, Liz Lichtenberger, Wendy Jones, Zona Lai, and Marie St. George

The rare, genetically based disorder, Williams syndrome (WMS), produces a constellation of distinctive cognitive, neuroanatomical, and electrophysiological features which we explore through the series of studies reported here. In this chapter, we focus primarily on the cognitive characteristics of WMS and begin to forge links among these characteristics, the brain, and the genetic basis of the disorder. The distinctive cognitive profile of individuals with WMS includes relative strengths in language and facial processing and profound impairment in spatial cognition. The cognitive profile of abilities, including what is 'typical' for individuals with WMS is discussed, but we also highlight areas of variability across the group of individuals with WMS that we have studied. Although the overall cognitive abilities (IQs) of individuals with WMS are typically in the mild-to-moderate range of mental retardation, the peaks and valleys within different cognitive domains make this syndrome especially intriguing to study across levels. Understanding the brain basis (and ultimately the genetic basis) for higher cognitive functioning is the goal we have begun to undertake with this line of interdisciplinary research.

Introduction

Crystal, an ambitious 14-year-old, was overheard to say "You're looking at a professional book writer. My books will be filled with drama, action, and excitement. Everyone will want to read them. I'm going to write books, page after page, stack after stack." Crystal is quite good at creating original stories on a moment's notice, most recently spinning a tale about a chocolate princess who saves her chocolate kingdom from melting by changing the color of the sun. Remarkably, her creative talents are not limited to storytelling, but extend to music as well; she has composed the lyrics and music to a song. Considering her ease with language, her creative ideas, and her unshaking enthusiasm, her ambition to become a writer may seem plausible—however, Crystal has an IQ of 49. She fails all Piagetian seriation and conservation tasks, milestones normally attained by age 8. She has reading, writing, and math skills comparable to those of a first-grader, demonstrates visuo-spatial abilities of a 5-year-old, and cannot be left alone without a babysitter.

Crystal has Williams syndrome (WMS), a rare (1 in 25,000) genetically based neurodevelopmental disorder. Characteristics of the syndrome include specific face and physical features; a variety of cardiovascular difficulties, including supravalvular aortic stenosis (SVAS); failure to thrive in infancy; transient-neonatal hypercalcemia; delayed language and motor development; and abnormal sensitivities to certain classes of sounds (hyperacusis) (Lenhoff, Wang, Greenberg, & Bellugi, 1997; Marriage & Scientist, 1995; Bellugi & Morris, 1995). The precise genetic underpinnings of WMS are becoming clear and are currently known to involve a submicroscopic deletion of one copy of about 20 contiguous genes on chromosome 7, including the gene for elastin (Korenberg et al., chap. 6; Frangiskakis et al., 1996).

Work being performed in our lab and others is mapping out the cognitive profile of WMS and its distinctive identifying features (Mervis, Morris, Bertrand, & Robinson, 1999; Karmiloff-Smith, 1998; Volterra, Capirci, Pezzini, Sabbadini, & Vicari, 1996; Bellugi, Bihrle, Neville, Jernigan, & Doherty, 1992; Bellugi, Wang, & Jernigan, 1994; Bellugi, Hickok, Jones, & Jernigan, 1996a; Bellugi, Klima, & Wang, 1996b; Bellugi & Wang, 1998; Bellugi, Lichtenberger, Mills, Galaburda, & Karenberg, 1999a, among others). Interest in Williams syndrome arises from the uneven cognitive profile that is associated with the syndrome through these studies, including specific dissociations in cognitive functions. In this chapter, we will review a series of formal and informal studies of cognitive behavior of individuals with Williams syndrome, largely from our laboratory over the past decade.

In this book, results are described across an array of disciplines from cognitive neuroscience to molecular genetics. This chapter and the next (Jones et al., chap. 2) sketch out some of the findings from studies of neurocognitive and social behavior in the same set of Williams individuals. Other chapters involve studies using brain-imaging techniques including event-related potentials (Mills et al., chap. 3) and magnetic-resonance imaging (Reiss et al., chap. 4) with the same subjects. The studies include brain cytoarchitectonics (Galaburda & Bellugi, chap. 5) as well as molecular genetics (Korenberg et al., chap. 6). The special strength of the program project is that (except for the cytoarchitectonic studies), the same subjects undergo cognitive, neurophysiological, neuromorphological, and molecular genetic probes. In this way, we can begin to link phenotype and genotype, as well as to link variability at one level with variability at other levels, in a large group of well-defined subjects. The chapters in this special issue show the linkages among cognitive, neurobiological, phenotypic, and genotypic profiles in order to create an initial picture of the functional neuroarchitecture of the syndrome. This linking occurs in several ways. By drawing on known connections between neurobiological systems and cognitive functions, we have begun to match cognitive abnormalities with their probable bases in neurobiological abnormalities. In addition, individual variation within the WMS population can be capitalized upon by predicting correlations between the strength of neurophysiological markers (in terms of event related potentials—ERPs) and performance on specific behavioral measures. Distinctive profile characteristics at the neurophysiological level (such as abnormal neurophysiological responses to face and language processing) can inform and refine our picture of aspects of the cognitive profile. Finally, we can take initial steps in the process of linking the presence or absence of copies of a small set of specific genes to the development of brain structure and function as well as to the specific cognitive profile of WMS.

Subjects

The groups of subjects with WMS who participated in the studies reported here involve a database of about 100 clinically and genetically diagnosed individuals with Williams syndrome, and are compared with Down Syndrome (DNS) individuals and normal controls, as well as with other specific disorders. Adolescent and adult individuals with WMS or DNS are part of a Program Project at The Salk Institute from the National Institute of Child Health and Human Development, "Williams Syndrome: Bridging Cognition and Gene." Infants and young children are part of a collaborative project with the Center for Neurodevelopmental studies at the University of California—San Diego (National Institute of Neurological Diseases and Stroke; and National Institute of Deafness and Other Communication Disorders). These studies include not only children with WMS or DNS syndrome, but also other projects including children with early onset focal lesions to the right or to the left hemisphere, with language impairment or autism. Subjects from the NICHD Program Project range in age from 10 and up and those from the Center for Neurodevelopmental studies range in age from birth to 10 years. Subjects are recruited for the WMS studies through our extensive contacts with families, the Williams Syndrome Association, national and regional conferences, private physicians, geneticists, cardiologists, and others that are familiar with the research in our laboratory. All are thoroughly screened prior to induction into the study and must pass a set of clear inclusionary and exclusionary criteria. Information about each subject's medical history is obtained from medical records, including a medical genetic evaluation confirming the diagnosis of WMS. In addition, a diagnostic interview, which tests for the common phenotypic features of the syndrome, is conducted with each subject and his/her caregiver. As part of this interview, a Diagnostic Score sheet (developed by the Medical Advisory Board of the Williams Syndrome Association) is completed (see Table 1.1 for a summary of some of the major diagnostic medical characteristics of WMS).

Molecular genetic testing (fluorescence *in situ* hybridization, or FISH) can now be used to confirm the deletion of one copy of the elastin gene and other surrounding genes in a small region of chromosome 7, characteristic of nearly all individuals with clinically diagnosed WMS. The studies in this paper and in subsequent papers in this volume (Jones et al., chap. 2; Korenberg et al., chap. 6; Mills et al., chap. 3; Reiss et al., chap. 4) include subjects who meet all aspects of our strict screening and diagnostic

Table 1.1
Summary of Major Williams Syndrome Medical Features

Neurological	*Facial Features*
average IQ 55 (range 40–90)	full prominent lips
poor coordination	stellate iris pattern
hypersensitivity to sound	prominent ear lobes
hoarse voice	wide mouth
Cardiovascular	small, widely spaced teeth
supervalvular aortic stenosis	medial eyebrow flare
peripheral pulmonary artery stenosis	flat nasal bridge
pulmonic valvular stenosis	short nose/anteverted nares
ventricular/atrial septal defects	*Other*
	elastin deletion probe (FISH)
	transient infantile hypercalcemia
	developmental delay (infants height and weight < 5th percentile)

criteria for Williams or Down syndrome and, importantly, the same individuals undergo probes at these major levels.

Throughout these studies of children and adults with WMS, we report on a variety of comparison groups: Normal individuals who are variously matched with WMS individuals on chronological age, mental age, or language age, and individuals with DNS who are matched in age and Full Scale IQ to the WMS group. As contrasts to the WMS data, we additionally report data from infants or young children with language impairment, with early focal lesions, and individuals with autism. The majority of the initial results we report in this paper consist of data collected from WMS subjects and from those with DNS, the latter primarily as a comparison group, matched in age and IQ, as well as normal controls matched for chronological age or mental age. Williams and Down groups were chosen initially because both are genetically based disorders resulting in mental retardation, but other comparison groups are important as well.

General Cognitive Functioning

Across an array of standardized conceptual and problem-solving tasks (some verbal, some nonverbal in nature), subjects with WMS demonstrate a consistent, serious impairment in general cognitive functioning. On general cognitive tasks such as IQ probes, most individuals with WMS rank in the 'mild-to-moderate mentally retarded' range, with global standard scores on IQ tests ranging from 40 to 90 and a mean of around 55 (Bellugi et al., 1996b). Figure 1.1 contrasts the distribution of Wechsler Full Scale IQ (Wechsler, 1974; Wechsler, 1981) of 82 subjects with WMS, with a typical nor-

Distribution of IQs in Williams Syndrome

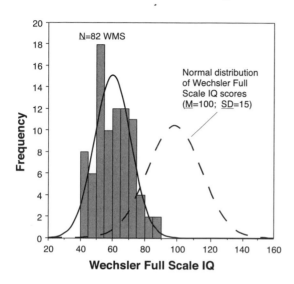

Figure 1.1
Wechsler Full Scale IQs in WMS range from 40 to 90, and are fairly normally distributed, with a mean IQ of approximately 55 (*SD* = 11).

mal distribution of Full Scale IQ scores. We can now describe what is "average" or "typical" and what is the distribution for WMS individuals on many standardized tests. As seen in the range of performance on IQ tests shown in Figure 1.1, there is also some variability within WMS as a group, with the WMS group mean shifted downward from the normal distribution into the mild-to-moderate range of mental retardation. Reflecting the variability in cognitive functioning, some adults with WMS live independently or semi-independently (Udwin, 1990), while others need significant help. It should be noted that arithmetic is an area of great difficulty for most individuals with WMS, but some are able to master addition and, in a small number of cases, subtraction and division as well. Reading is a challenge for some, while others have been noted to be avid readers of books, magazines, and newspapers, but often on very specific topics of interest (Howlin, Davies, & Udwin, 1998).

The typical global cognitive impairment that is seen in WMS is similar to that found in DNS in our studies. As shown in Figure 1.2, adolescents with WMS and those with DNS in our studies score equally poorly across the board on IQ tests such as the Wechsler Intelligence Scale for Children—Revised (WISC-R; Wechsler, 1974) or Wechsler

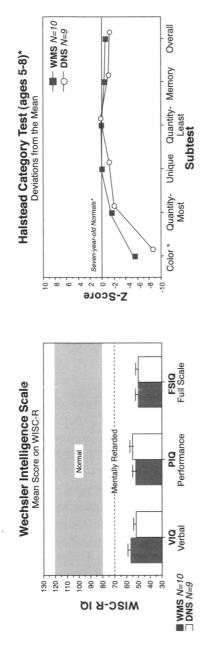

Figure 1.2
Subjects with WMS and DNS consistently score below 'normal' on tests of general cognitive ability, such as the WISC-R (Wechsler Intelligence Test for Children—Revised) (left) and the Halstead Category Test (right).

Adult Intelligence Scale—Revised (WAIS-R; Wechsler, 1981). In each of these subject groups, there was no clinically significant difference between Verbal and Performance IQ scores on the Wechsler scales. In addition, both groups showed equal degrees of impairment on cognitive probes such as the Halstead Reitan Neuropsychological Battery (Reitan & Wolfson, 1985), and general tests of conceptual knowledge, information, or math achievement, and Piagetian tests of conservation, including conservation of number, weight, and substance (Bellugi et al., 1992; Bellugi et al., 1994; Bellugi et al., 1996b).

Adolescents and adults with WMS have been found to have a conceptual understanding of basic biological categories of living things such as people, animals, and plants, that is only equivalent to that of normal 6-year-olds (Carey, 1985). The limited biological knowledge and understanding of subjects with WMS is also evident in their failure to attain the level of conceptual restructuring that most normal children achieve by age 10 or 11 (Johnson & Carey, 1998; Rossen, Klima, Bellugi, Bihrle, & Jones, 1996). For example, adolescents and adults with WMS have difficulty differentiating *not alive* into the conceptual categories of *dead, inanimate, unreal, or nonexistent*. A specific example of the limits of conceptual knowledge in WMS is from a reported instance of a 21-year-old woman with WMS (Verbal IQ of 69) who was literate and read several books on her favorite topic: Vampires. When this subject was asked what a vampire is, she responded reasonably and clearly that a vampire is "a man who climbs into ladies' bedrooms at night and sinks his teeth into their necks." When asked why vampires do that, she thought for a bit, and then said, "Vampires must have an inordinate fondness for necks" (Johnson & Carey, 1998).

Along with their general cognitive deficits, individuals with WMS typically have difficulty in mathematics and its application to everyday life, such as making change, balancing a checkbook, and cooking from recipes. In our studies, many individuals with WMS would rather receive 50 pennies than five dollars as a reward. These difficulties are in keeping with their difficulties in mastering Piagetian conservation. Another probe, the Cognitive Estimation Test, assessed WMS subjects' abilities to estimate length, weight, and similar concepts (Dehaene, 1997). The test was administered to 10 adolescents and adults with WMS. Many responses to the questions asked in this task were very far off the mark. For example, when asked, "What is the length of a dollar bill?," a 15-year-old subject with WMS responded, "five feet"; an 18-year-old subject with WMS responded, "four feet"; and a 20-year-old subject with WMS responded, "one inch." On another question, "What is the normal length of a bus?," individuals with WMS responded: "30 inches" (a 12-year-old); "3 inches or 100 inches maybe" (a 15-year-old); "2 inches, 10 feet" (a 24-year-old). Each of these examples shows the great difficulty that adolescents and even adults with WMS have in estimating values that are easily estimated by many younger, normally developing children (Kopera-Frye, Dehaene, & Streissguth, 1996).

Relatively Spared Expressive Language in Williams Syndrome

Considering the general cognitive impairment exhibited in WMS, their noticeable facility with complex language (albeit not always used correctly) often comes as a surprise to people who encounter individuals with this syndrome. Adolescents and adults with WMS tend to be articulate, and are talkative to the point of being loquacious. This relative strength is in contrast to the considerable linguistic deficits in individuals with DNS, who typically present with major deficits in syntax. We have investigated many facets of language processing in WMS. We briefly describe the development of language in the WMS population and then provide a brief overview of aspects of language: Grammar, lexical semantics, and narrative production.

Stages of Language Development   Although mature WMS linguistic performance shows that language is a major strength in the WMS cognitive profile and radically different from typical DNS, the initial stages of development do not clearly predict this. In older children and adolescents with WMS, linguistic abilities seem relatively preserved, whereas in older DNS individuals, linguistic abilities are far below those of WMS. Hence, in their mature state, the behavioral phenotypes of WMS and DNS test the outer limits of the dissociations that can occur between language and cognition.

How do these contrasting profiles come about? In our studies of younger children with WMS and DNS, we are pushing these two profiles back to their origins, seeking the point at which language and other aspects of cognition diverge over time. The behavioral phenotype of WMS undergoes dramatic change across the first years of life, starting out with extreme delay at all developmental milestones, including language, but with islands of sparing in the perception of sounds and faces. By uncovering differences between WMS and DNS syndrome children in the first stages of prespeech and language development, and comparing them with other populations, we can obtain insights into the factors responsible for the contrasting profiles of language and cognition displayed later in development.

ONSET OF WORDS.   The onset of first words was studied using a parental report of language acquisition, the MacArthur Communicative Development Inventory (CDI; Fenson et al., 1993), in a sample of 54 children with WMS and 39 children with DNS (ranging in age from 12 to 60 months). Surprisingly, there were no significant differences reported in the onset of first words between children with WMS and DNS (Singer-Harris, Bellugi, Bates, Jones, & Rossen, 1997). Although both groups were found to be equally and massively delayed as compared to normally developing chil-

Development of First Words in Young Children with Williams and Down Syndrome

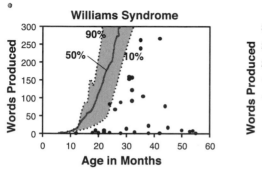

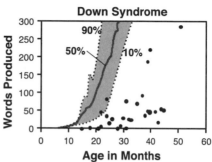

Figure 1.3
The total number of words produced by young children (infants and toddlers) on the MacArthur Communicative Development Inventory (CDI) for children with WMS (left) and DNS (right) shows considerable variability and equally delayed onset of words in both groups. Shaded area represents trajectories of normal children in a large study using the CDI.

dren at the initial stages (see Figure 1.3), differential patterns of language acquisition emerged. Relative to one another, children with DNS exhibited an early advantage for communicative gestures, while children with WMS displayed a strong advantage for grammar later in development. Moreover, there was a tendency for comprehension levels to be high relative to production in DNS and an opposite tendency in WMS infants and toddlers. Parents of DNS children reported that their children could understand many words but not produce them; parents of WMS children often reported the opposite: That their young WMS children could say many words they did not understand. A 4-year-old WMS child brought to the lab for testing could accurately repeat words such as 'encyclopedia' or 'Britannica' with clarity and precision, although investigation showed that she could not describe or even provide hints that she understood any aspect of the meaning of the words.

FROM FIRST WORDS TO GRAMMAR.   The next phase of development is characterized by dramatic changes in language in normal children and in WMS, including the rapid acquisition of basic morphosyntactic structures. In normal children, these events take place between 16 and 30 months of age. As grammar emerges, children with WMS in general improve dramatically, whereas children with DNS tend to plateau rather early in development, falling further and further behind. WMS young children then move ahead in grammar acquisition compared to DNS and, in fact, the linguistic phenotypes of the two groups diverge at the point where grammar is acquired and beyond, a provocative finding in view of the contrasting profiles that are observed later in life. In some ways, results suggest that DNS language comprehension has a delayed but relatively normal developmental pathway in infancy, whereas WMS language development may be more deviant from the outset (Karmiloff-Smith et al., 1997; Singer-Harris et al., 1997; Rossen et al., 1996).

Grammar The general cognitive impairment seen in adolescents and adults with WMS stands in stark contrast to their relative strength in language, their facility and ease in using sentences with complex syntax, not generally characteristic of other mentally retarded groups (Rossen et al., 1996). To assess their comprehension and use of complex syntax, several studies were conducted.

On tasks that measure grammatical abilities, adolescents and adults with WMS showed relatively strong abilities compared with DNS. For example, on a task of comprehension of passive sentences, subjects had to choose which of four pictures best fit the meaning of the sentence, such as "the horse is chased by the man." The sentences in the study were semantically reversible passives, such that "the man is chased by the horse" is also a well-formed grammatical sentence. Therefore, since either the horse or the man can do the chasing, to correctly perform the task, the subject must have an understanding of the underlying syntax of the sentence. Adolescents with WMS showed relatively strong performance compared to DNS who performed close to chance (Bellugi, Bihrle, Jernigan, Trauner, & Doherty, 1990; Bellugi et al., 1996b).

On several other syntax tests, subjects with WMS scored significantly higher than subjects with DNS: (a) the Test for Reception of Grammar (TROG; Bishop, 1982), (b) the Kempler Test of Syntax (Kempler & VanLanker, 1993), (c) the Curtiss-Yamada Comprehensive Language Evaluation (CYCLE; Curtiss & Yamada, 1988), and (d) the Clinical Evaluation of Language Fundamentals (CELF; Semel, Wiig, & Secord, 1987). On a probe of detection of syntactic and semantic anomalies (Dennis & Whitaker, 1976), again the WMS group scored significantly higher than the DNS group. The ability to detect and correct anomalies in the syntax of a sentence may depend on the knowledge of syntactic constraints and the ability to reflect upon grammatical form. Some of these are metalinguistic abilities that, in normal children, are mastered considerably after the acquisition of grammar. These skills are more fully developed in WMS than in DNS. In addition, the spontaneous language production of adolescents and adults with WMS shows that they typically produce a variety of grammatically complex forms, including passive sentences, conditional clauses, and embedded relative clauses, although there are occasional morpho-syntactic errors, and even some systematic ones, e.g., in language about spatial relations (Karmiloff-Smith, 1998; Lichtenberger & Bellugi, 1998; Rubba & Klima, 1991).

Excellent Processing of Conditionals by Individuals
with Williams Syndrome

Conditionals Task

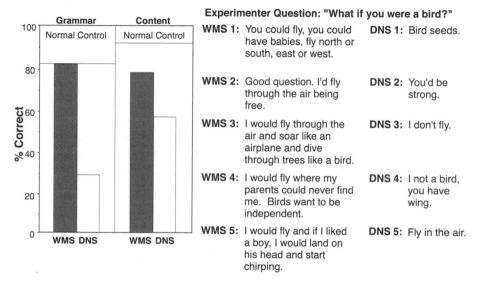

Experimenter Question: "What if you were a bird?"

WMS 1: You could fly, you could have babies, fly north or south, east or west.

DNS 1: Bird seeds.

WMS 2: Good question. I'd fly through the air being free.

DNS 2: You'd be strong.

WMS 3: I would fly through the air and soar like an airplane and dive through trees like a bird.

DNS 3: I don't fly.

WMS 4: I would fly where my parents could never find me. Birds want to be independent.

DNS 4: I not a bird, you have wing.

WMS 5: I would fly and if I liked a boy, I would land on his head and start chirping.

DNS 5: Fly in the air.

Figure 1.4
Individuals with WMS (12 years and older) perform significantly better than those with DNS (age- and Full Scale IQ-matched to WMS subjects) on syntactic processing tasks (e.g., conditional sentences) on both grammar and content. Examples of responses by subjects with WMS and DNS are shown. Normal control levels are shown by a line.

Individuals with WMS display a stronger ability to process conditional questions ("What would you do if . . .") than individuals with DNS (Figure 1.4). In a sample of 14 subjects, half with WMS and half with DNS, the individuals with WMS responded correctly to the conditional questions 83% of the time, while the individuals with DNS responded correctly only 29% of the time ($t = 4.03$; $p < .01$). Teens and adults with WMS tended to respond in complete sentences whose content indicated they understood the question and, importantly, tended to respond with the appropriate grammatical marking. For example, when subjects were asked questions such as "What if you were a bird?," responses included: "I would fly through the air and soar like an airplane and dive through trees like a bird and land like a bird," "I would fly where my parents could never find me. Birds want to be independent," and "I would fly and if I liked a boy, I would land on his head and start chirping." These types of responses were in contrast to those of the subjects with DNS which included sentence fragments, such as "fly in the air," and included content sometimes indicating that the question might have been misunderstood, such as "bird seeds."

Lexical Semantics   Although individuals with WMS demonstrate considerable linguistic abilities given their level of other cognitive abilities, even to the naive ear, aspects of their language—particularly their vocabulary—sometimes strike people as unusual. One of the first groups of WMS we studied was referred by a cardiologist who asked if there was interest in studying a group of individuals with a heart defect who "talked funny." In casual conversation with WMS individuals, one may notice that they sometimes use unusual, rather sophisticated words—unexpected, considering their overall level of cognitive functioning (e.g., "commentator," "sauté," "mince," and "alleviate"). Sometimes, these words are used correctly, but other times they are partially, but not completely, appropriate in the accompanying context. For example, one subject stated "I have to evacuate the glass" as she emptied a glass of water. The transitive verb 'evacuate' conveys emptying something, but most often this refers to removing people from something that is containing them, as in 'evacuate the city'. The erroneous word choices are often in the right semantic field, but they sometimes fail to convey semantic nuances appropriate for the context.

Across a realm of studies, WMS individuals appear to show a *proclivity* for unusual words, not typical of normal or DNS subjects. Despite their low IQ scores, adolescents with WMS were typically correct in matching such words as 'canine,' 'abrasive,' and 'solemn' with a picture on the Peabody Vocabulary test; note that WMS score higher than their mental age on that test, whereas DNS score lower than their mental age (Figure 1.5a). In a task of semantic organization, subjects were asked to name all the animals they could think of in a minute. WMS subjects not only gave significantly more responses than mental-age matched normal controls, some also produced more uncommon animal names than DNS subjects or control subjects (Rossen et al., 1996; Wang & Bellugi, 1993). For example, one WMS subject said in sequence, "tiger, owl, sea lion, zebra, hippopotamus, turtle, lizard, reptile, frog, beaver, giraffe, chihuahua," and another said, ". . . ibex, whale, bull, yak, zebra, puppy, kitten, tiger, koala, dragon." Many of the DNS subjects, in contrast, repeated animals or included nonanimals in their responses; for example, one DNS individual said, "goats, rabbits, bunnies, horsey, french fries . . ." (see Figure 1.5b). Some important developmental trends have been noted in the within-category naming abilities of individuals with WMS (Rossen et al., 1996). For example, in a sample of 84 individuals with WMS from 5 to 40 years who were administered the semantic-fluency task, age-related increases were noted in performance; there was a significant positive correlation between production of words and age ($r = .34$, $p < .001$) with a steep rise around the age of 11 (Figure 1.5c).

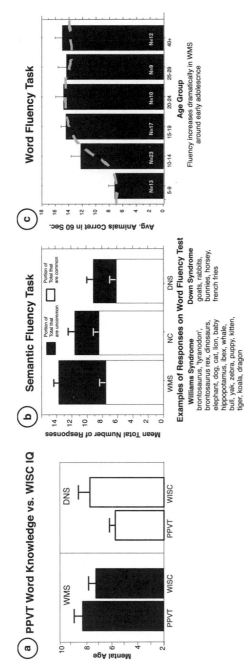

Figure 1.5

(a) Although the WMS and DNS subjects had comparably low IQ scores, WMS subjects scored significantly higher than their mental age on a probe that taps lexical knowledge, whereas DNS scores significantly lower than their mental age. (b) On a semantic-fluency task requiring subjects to produce as many names as possible in 60 sec, WMS adolescents produce far more responses than the DNS group; in fact, as many as mental age matched normal controls. WMS also produced significantly more uncommon words than their DNS counterparts or than the matched controls. (c) On the semantic-fluency test, there is a steady rise in the numbers of examples from WMS across the age span from 5 to 40 years; in particular, there is a sharp increase in fluency around the age of 11.

To gain insight into the nature of semantic organization, individuals with WMS, DNS, and fourth-grade normal controls were given a series of experimental probes to investigate their processing of homonyms, words with more than one meaning. These tasks examine the relative salience of primary (higher frequency) and secondary (lower frequency) meanings of homonyms, such as SWALLOW (gulp, bird); WATCH (to look, time); FEET (toes, measure). We constructed the list of homonyms chosen so that one meaning (the primary meaning) was more common than the other meaning (the secondary meaning), according to comprehensive norms (Rossen et al., 1996). Three tasks were performed using the homonyms: Free association, similarity judgment, and definitions. The free-association task required the participants to say the first word that came to mind after hearing a homonym. In this task, all three groups responded similarly, offering associates related to the primary meaning of the homonym.

In the similarity-judgment task, subjects were presented with word triads composed of the homonym, and words related to the primary and secondary meanings (Rossen et al., 1996; example shown in Figure 1.6a). Subjects were asked to repeat the word triad after the experimenter and then pick which two words "go together best." Normal controls tended to choose the primary meanings more frequently than secondary meanings as did the subjects with DNS. Subjects with WMS, in contrast, provided an equal number of primary and secondary meanings, suggesting anomalous semantic organization (see Figure 1.6b).

For the definitions task, subjects were asked to "tell me everything you know about what (the homonym) means." If the subject did not provide both meanings spontaneously, the experimenter probed for another meaning: "Can you tell me anything else that (the homonym) means?" WMS were just as likely as controls to provide definitions compatible with the primary meaning of the homonyms. However, just as in the similarity-judgment task, they were also significantly more likely than controls or DNS to provide, in addition, definitions compatible with the secondary meaning of the homonym (see Figure 1.6c). Taken together, the data from the similarity-judgment task and the definitions task suggest that there may be some unusual aspects to semantic processing in WMS involving, perhaps, attenuation of the usual effect of frequency or familiarity (Rossen et al., 1996).

There is other related evidence to suggest unusual semantic processing in individuals with WMS. Event-related brain potentials (ERPs) were recorded during auditory sentence comprehension (Mills, Neville, Appelbaum, Prat, & Bellugi, 1997). Subjects heard sentences that included a semantic anomaly, such as "I have five fingers on my moon." The semantic anomaly "moon" instead of the expected word "hand" evoked the N400 component of the waveform. Analysis of the N400 showed that the WMS subjects did not produce the typical scalp distribution found in normal subjects, but

Anomalous Semantic Processing in Williams Syndrome: Homonyms Task

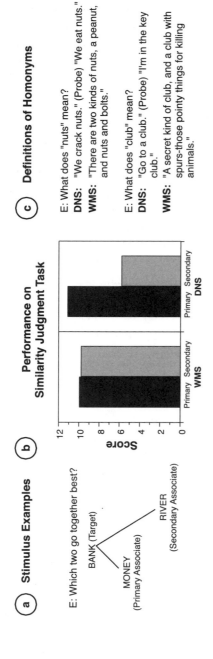

(a) Stimulus Examples

E: Which two go together best?

BANK (Target)

MONEY (Primary Associate)

RIVER (Secondary Associate)

(b) Performance on Similarity Judgment Task

Score: 0, 2, 4, 6, 8, 10, 12

WMS: Primary, Secondary

DNS: Primary, Secondary

(c) Definitions of Homonyms

E: What does "nuts" mean?
DNS: "We crack nuts." (Probe) "We eat nuts."
WMS: "There are two kinds of nuts, a peanut, and nuts and bolts."

E: What does "club" mean?
DNS: "Go to a club." (Probe) "I'm in the key club."
WMS: "A secret kind of club, and a club with spurs-those pointy things for killing animals."

Figure 1.6

(a) The figure shows stimulus examples of homonyms task with primary and secondary meanings (e.g., 'bank'). (b) Subjects with DNS and normal mental age controls provide more primary meanings than secondary meanings of the homonyms, as would be expected. Subjects with WMS, in contrast, provide an equal number of primary and secondary meanings, suggesting anomolous semantic organization. (c) Sample responses show that WMS subjects are able to access both the primary and secondary meanings of homonyms while DNS subjects access only one meaning, sometimes with two responses. For the meaning of 'club,' a DNS individual said "Go to a club" and then "I'm in the key club" whereas a WMS individual said: "A secret kind of club, and a club with spurs . . ."

rather, showed a more distributed N400 response, not the right-greater-than-left asymmetry typical of normal subjects. This finding may be related to the unusual semantic proclivities shown by WMS in the tasks described above. Furthermore, the neural systems underlying syntactic processing may also turn out to be different from normal, despite the relative sparing of language abilities in WMS subjects compared to DNS (Mills, 1998; see also Mills et al., chap. 3).

Comparison of Language in WMS with Other Contrast Groups   In our studies, we have had the opportunity to contrast aspects of language development across diverse groups of subjects, ages 4–12, as part of a project with the Center for Neurodevelopmental Studies, to gain a fuller understanding of language abilities in children with WMS. On a sentence-repetition task, the Carrow Elicited Language Inventory (CELI; Carrow, 1974), we compared children with WMS ($N = 29$) to children who were classified as language impaired ($N = 24$) and to children with early focal brain lesions ($N = 14$), as well as to 86 normal control children. The language impaired children were defined as those with Wechsler Performance IQs of 80 or better, but whose scores were at least 1.5 standard deviations below the mean on a standardized test of language production. All four groups showed clear progress in language development across the age range (including the children with WMS who, in contrast, show no development on cognitive tests such as Piagetian tests of conservation). The WMS group repeated significantly fewer sentences correctly (59.6%) than did the normal group (84.8%) ($F(1,113) = 28.73$, $p < .0001$). However, the performance of individuals with WMS was *not* significantly different from that of children who were language impaired or who had focal brain lesions (see Figure 1.7a). This is of interest because there was no global cognitive impairment in the language impaired or focal lesion groups, yet subjects with WMS, this genetically based group of mentally retarded individuals, performed at a level on this language task that was comparable to that of these contrast groups.

In another comparison using a sentence-repetition task, groups of children with WMS ($N = 68$) and a small number of children with DNS ($N = 11$), who were functioning at about the same level of general cognitive ability, were contrasted with normal controls ($N = 59$). The number of morphosyntactic errors in the sentences across the age span was examined for each group (Figure 1.7b). Normally developing subjects showed a decreasing number of errors from ages 2 to 8 years and obtained a nearly perfect score between ages 8 and 9, on average. Similar to the developmental trends mentioned earlier, subjects with WMS also showed clear developmental progress on this task, although slower than normal, with a decreasing number of morphosyntactic errors from ages 4 to 14 and, on average, were making few errors by ages 14–16 years. In contrast, the subjects with DNS showed a significant amount of variability in their per-

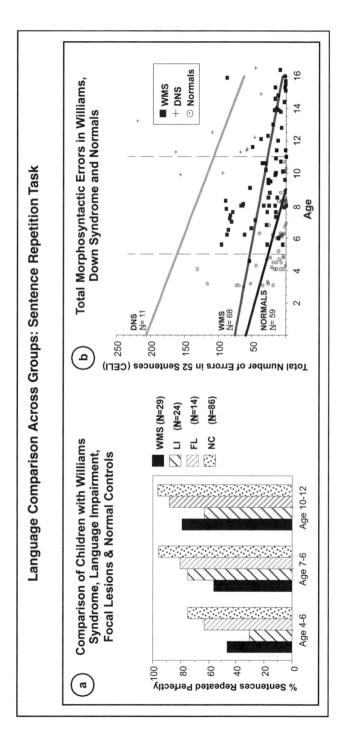

Figure 1.7

(a) Children with WMS, children with early focal lesions, and children with language impairment are not significantly different from one another in their ability to correctly repeat sentences at all ages. (b) The number of morphological errors made during the sentence-repetition task in a group of children with WMS, with DNS, and a group of normally developing children. The number of errors decreases consistently from ages 5 to 16 in children with WMS, which is similar to a developmental trend seen in normals at a younger age.

formance with a decreasing number of morphosyntactic errors as they progressed through early childhood into adolescence, but they continued to exhibit errors in performance through age 16.

In summary, across a variety of language tasks, the subjects with WMS perform far better than age- and IQ-matched individuals with DNS and, in a direct language comparison, perform similarly to subjects with language impairment without mental retardation or subjects who have had early focal lesions (Bellugi, Losh, Reilly, & Anderson, 1998). Although subjects with WMS typically start with a delay in the production of first words that is equal to that of subjects with DNS, by adolescence and adulthood, language is clearly a relative strength of WMS; thus, the early stages of language do not predict the later ones. The distribution of abilities across the major domains consisting of language and visuo-spatial abilities in WMS can be seen in Figure 1.8, which shows scores across more than 100 individuals with WMS for a standardized vocabulary test, the Peabody Picture Vocabulary Test—Revised (PPVT-R; Dunn & Dunn, 1981) and a standardized task that requires copying geometric shapes, the Developmental Test of Visual-Motor Integration (VMI; Beery, 1997). The contrast between performance in the two domains, language and spatial abilities, is striking. Whereas lexical abilities in WMS individuals on the PPVT-R are higher than their mental age, see also Figure 1.5a), visuo-spatial abilities are markedly low across individuals with WMS of all ages. As we discuss next, this pattern of performance in WMS is opposite that of individuals with DNS.

Controversial Issues in Language and Cognition As interest in WMS has grown, the number of studies has rapidly increased. Controversial issues have been raised by the research on WMS, some having to do with the relation between language and other aspects of cognition, which continue to be a matter of debate (Clahsen & Almazan, 1998; Bates, 1997; Karmiloff-Smith et al., 1997; Stevens & Karmiloff-Smith, 1997; Levy, 1996; Pinker, 1994; Pinker, 1997). Some consider the syndrome as a good example of the modularity of language as a system separate in significant respects from other general cognitive abilities. Others argue that since adults with WMS have been found to function in relevant ways at the level of 5- to 7-year-olds, that level would provide a sufficient substrate of cognitive abilities for the development of complex syntax and, accordingly, WMS does not represent a dissociation between language and general cognitive functions. Levy (1996) argues that there may be "uniquely preserved accessing privileges for language which may enable individuals with WMS to reach levels of performance that they cannot reach through other modalities." There are unresolved questions about the relationship between syntax and semantics, about the intactness of levels of language in WMS. Yet, most researchers generally agree that the structural as-

Distribution of Language and Spatial Measures in Williams Syndrome

(a)   **Language Vocabulary Scores**

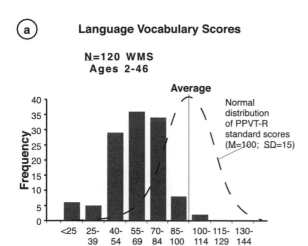

N=120 WMS
Ages 2-46

Peabody Picture Vocabulary Test, Revised (PPVT-R) Standard Score

(b)   **Visual-Spatial Scores**

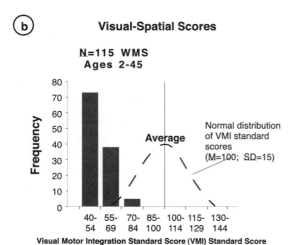

N=115 WMS
Ages 2-45

Visual Motor Integration Standard Score (VMI) Standard Score

Figure 1.8
(a) On the Peabody Picture Vocabulary Test—Revised (PPVT-R), the WMS group shows a distribution in performance with some subjects performing in the normal range. (b) On the Developmental Test of Visual–Motor Integration (VMI), the WMS group shows significantly worse performance in their visual-motor skills in contrast to their lexical knowledge. Most subjects, regardless of age, score on the floor of the spatial task.

pects of language (e.g., morphology and syntax) are a relative strength in WMS, perhaps different from other syndromes that involve mental retardation (Bellugi & Wang, 1998; Karmiloff-Smith, 1998; Volterra et al., 1996).

The Intersection of Language and Affect   A distinctive facet of the language abilities of individuals with WMS is their ability to use their considerable linguistic skills to engage others socially (Bellugi et al., 1996b). Many individuals with WMS display a strong impulse toward interpersonal contact and a proclivity for affective expression, although their social behavior is not always appropriate (Einfeld, Tonge, & Florio, 1997). The intersection of language and social behavior in individuals with WMS has been investigated through a series of narrative tasks in which subjects are asked to 'tell' a story from a series of static images in a wordless picture book (Bellugi & Wang, 1998; Bellugi et al., 1998; Bellugi, Mills, Jernigan, Hickok, & Galaburda, 1999b). The following paper (Jones et al., chap. 2) provides examples of the affectively expressive language used by subjects with WMS compared to subjects with DNS. The most obvious characteristic differentiating subjects with WMS from those with DNS and age-matched normal controls is in their use of narrative enrichment devices during this story-telling task. The information conveyed by the enrichment devices goes beyond what is explicitly presented in the static pictures themselves. By linguistic means (through choice of words and use of prosody), the emotions and thoughts of the characters pictured are expressed, and also the emotions and evaluations of the 'narrator'—in this case, the particular WMS individual.

As will be shown in the next paper, individuals with WMS show an abundance of affectivity in both prosody and lexical devices and appear to be able to manipulate affective linguistic devices for the purposes of storytelling. (Affective prosody was measured by noting how frequently paralinguistic affective expression was used, including pitch change, vocalic lengthening and modifications in volume.) Affectivity in lexical devices was measured in the frequency of exclamatory phrases and other devices to engage the audience (e.g., '*Suddenly splash*! The water came up'; '*Lo and behold*'). This pattern of increased linguistic affectivity was found to be strikingly different from what was found in subjects with DNS, as well as in normal individuals at any age or in the other contrast groups studied (e.g., individuals with early focal brain lesions and Language-Impaired children).

In sum, in adolescents and adults with WMS, language is typically used effectively (and sometimes effusively) in social situations. Perhaps, a prime characteristic of individuals with WMS is a strong impulse toward social contact and affective expression. Thus, the social and language profiles of individuals with WMS are also in striking contrast to individuals with other disorders such as autism.

The Domain of Spatial Cognition: Peaks and Valleys of Abilities

Unlike language, with its well-defined levels of phonology, morphology, syntax, and discourse, the domain of spatial cognition has largely resisted fractionation into components (c.f., Stiles-Davis, Kritchevsky, & Bellugi, 1988). By comparing the spatial cognitive deficits in WMS and DNS, we can examine different patterns that might emerge as a result of different genetic anomalies (Bellugi et al., 1990; Bellugi et al., 1992; Bellugi et al., 1999a; Bihrle, Bellugi, Delis, & Marks, 1989; Bihrle, 1990). A discussion of some of our specific findings follows.

Differing Patterns of Spatial Deficits in WMS vs. DNS   In order to explore spatial cognition, a battery of standardized tasks was administered to subjects with WMS and DNS. WMS subjects were found to be severely impaired on the Block Design subtest of the WISC-R (Wechsler, 1974), and on the VMI (Visuo-motor Integration, Beery, 1997). The Block Design task requires the subject to arrange a set of blocks (with sides colored red, white, and half-and-half) so they replicate increasingly complex stimulus patterns. The VMI task requires the individual to copy geometric shapes ranging from straight lines and triangles to more complex interpolated three-dimensional shapes. When subjects with WMS are asked to draw, whether copying an illustration or doing free drawing, the product typically has poor cohesion and lacks overall organization within the images. In other populations, important developmental trends have been noted on the VMI; individuals with prenatal focal lesions to the right hemisphere exhibit good recovery over time and improved performance on this task by age 8 years. In contrast, even into adulthood, individuals with WMS tend to plateau and remain basically at the level of normally developing 5-year-olds (Beret, Bellugi, Hickok, & Stiles, 1996). Frequently, we have noted WMS individuals verbally mediating their way through drawings, thus enabling us to add the individual's own verbal labels to interpret the components of the drawing (Figure 1.9). For example, drawings of houses by WMS individuals may show a door, a roof and windows, but the parts might be depicted in an unrecognizable relationship to each other (e.g., windows stretched out across the page outside of the boundaries of the house). In contrast, comparable subjects with DNS might produce drawings with little detail, but showing good closure and form, with appropriate relationships among the elements (see Figure 1.9, top). The illustration also shows drawings of a bicycle by individuals with WMS and with DNS both age 11, and both with IQs in the 50s (Bellugi, 1998). Note that the drawing of a bicycle by the individual with DNS is simple and lacks extensive detail, yet it is recognizable and has good closure and integrated form to the parts. In contrast, the drawing of a bicycle by the individual with WMS is highly fragmented; the pedals are off to one

Different Spatial Deficits in Drawing by WMS and DNS Children Matched on Age and IQ

Drawings of a House by Individuals with Williams and Down Syndrome

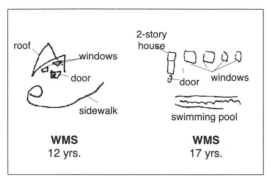

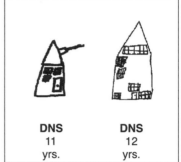

Drawings of a Bicycle by Individuals with Williams and Down Syndrome

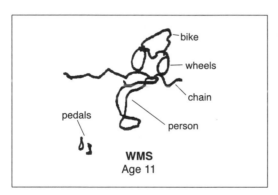

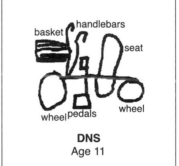

Figure 1.9
Free drawings of houses by age- and IQ-matched adolescents with WMS and DNS show different spatial deficits. The drawings by subjects with WMS contain many parts of houses but the parts are not organized coherently. In contrast, the DNS subjects' drawings are simplified but have the correct overall configuration of houses. Similarly, drawings of a bicycle by a subject with WMS shows the 'person' upside down, the pedals off to the side, and the chain floating in the air, all in a disorganized fashion (verbal labels were added by the subject as he drew). In contrast, the matched subject with DNS produces a simplified but recognizable drawing with the correct overall configuration of a bicycle.

Different Deficits in Block Design for Williams and Down:
(Fractionated Attention to Detail in Williams)

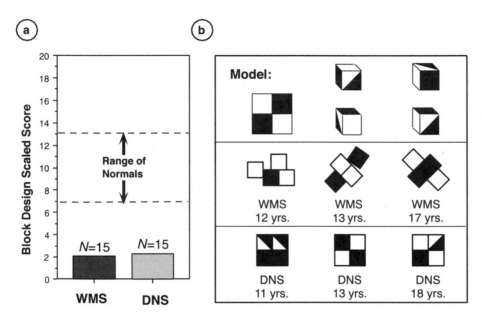

Figure 1.10
(a) On average, adolescents with WMS and DNS were similarly impaired on the WISC-R Block Design sub-test. (b) Although the end score is equally poor for WMS and DNS (scaled scores more than 2 SD below normal), they fail in very different ways. Subjects with WMS typically show disjointed and fragmented designs, while age- and IQ-matched DNS subjects tend to make errors in internal details while maintaining the overall configuration.

side, the person is upside down, and the chain is floating in the air (see Figure 1.9, bottom).

In a study using the Block Design subtest of the WISC-R (Wechsler, 1974), spatial-cognitive deficits were found in subjects with both WMS and DNS, with equally poor levels of performance (WMS $N = 15$; DNS $N = 15$). However, examination of the *process* by which they arrived at their scores reveals striking differences between the two syndromes (Bellugi et al., 1996b; Bellugi et al., 1999b; Wang, Doherty, Rourke, & Bellugi, 1995). Although they failed to provide correct designs, the subjects with DNS generally kept the global configuration of the block arrangements, with details of the internal configurations of the designs incorrect. Subjects with WMS, by contrast, failed

Differential Impairment on a Local/Global Processing Task in Williams and Down Syndrome

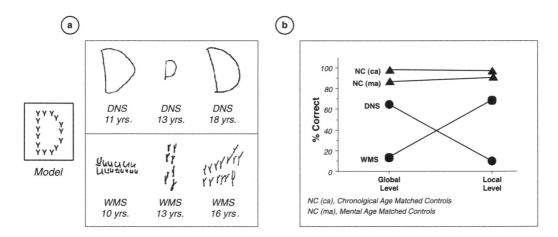

Figure 1.11
(a) On the Delis Hierarchical Processing task, subjects are asked to copy a large global figure made of smaller local forms (e.g., a 'D' made out of 'Y's). Both groups fail but in significantly different ways: Subjects with WMS tend to produce the local elements sprinkled across the page, whereas age- and IQ-matched DNS subjects tend to produce only the global forms. (b) When drawing these designs from memory or from copy, subjects with WMS tend to reproduce the local level of the stimuli with more accuracy, subjects with DNS tend to reproduce the global level of the stimuli with more accuracy. Normal chronological age-matched subjects reproduce both levels of the figure with approximately equal accuracy.

to keep the global configuration of the designs, appearing biased toward the details of the designs (see Figure 1.10). They frequently placed the blocks in apparently haphazard, noncontiguous arrangements. In a process analysis comparing adolescents with WMS and DNS, those with WMS were found to make far more moves, and very frequently made these moves in continuously fragmented patterns. Thus, across several spatial-cognitive tasks (copying drawings, free drawings, block design), there are marked and specific spatial deficits that have been found in WMS (Bellugi, 1998).

Seeing the Forest or the Trees   To investigate and characterize these various visual-cognitive impairments, an experimental task that distinguishes two levels of structure, involving both local and global features in a balanced array was used. Items were composed of local components that together constituted a global form (i.e., a big 'D' made up of little 'Y's). On these tasks, characteristic deficits that separated the subjects with WMS from those with DNS were found (Bihrle et al., 1989). When asked to draw the designs made of two levels of hierarchical structure, both groups failed, but in distinctively different ways. In these paradigms, subjects with WMS typically produced primarily the local forms sprinkled across the page, and were impaired at producing the global forms. Subjects with DNS showed the opposite pattern; they tended to produce the global forms without including the local forms (see Figure 1.11). This was true whether subjects had to reproduce forms from memory (after a 5-sec delay) or whether they were asked to copy the forms that lay in front of them. In a follow-up study using a larger number of subjects with WMS (N = 35), WMS subjects were again found to show more of a bias toward the local level of the stimuli than to the global level ($p <$ .01). In perceptual-matching tasks as well, using hierarchical figures, subjects with WMS showed a distinct local bias. These results suggest differential processing patterns in WMS and DNS, and highlight what may be a bias toward fractionation of the gestalt and over attention to detail, at the expense of the whole (Atkinson, King, Braddick, & Nokes, 1997; Wang et al., 1995; Bihrle et al., 1989; Bellugi et al., 1999a).

Face Processing: An Island of Sparing in WMS   Despite their severe spatial-cognitive dysfunctions, there are domains in which subjects with WMS display selective sparing of abilities. Subjects with WMS demonstrate a remarkable ability to recognize, discriminate, and remember unfamiliar and familiar faces (Rossen, Jones, Wang, & Klima, 1995a). However, this ability was not noted in individuals with DNS. In fact, the performance of the WMS group is at a near-normal level (Jones, Hickok, & Lai, 1998a; Rossen, Smith, Jones, Bellugi, & Korenberg, 1995b). These strengths include abilities related to the perception of faces, such as the ability to recognize faces when seen in various lighting conditions and orientations. Across an array of tasks involving faces, individuals with WMS outperform those with DNS (Jones et al., 1998a; see Figure 1.12). The Benton Test of Facial Recognition (Benton, Hamsher, Varney, & Spreen, 1983b) is a face-discrimination task in which subjects are asked to identify which ones of six faces match the target individual. The faces involve the same individual under different conditions of lighting, shadow, and orientation. The Warrington Recognition Memory Test (Warrington, 1984) is a recognition-memory task that presents the subject with unfamiliar faces. The Mooney Closure Task (Mooney, 1957) is considered a closure task in which black and white photographs of faces are shown with many background and facial details ablated by shading. Subjects are required to decide whether the face is a male or female or whether it is someone young or old. In separate studies using the Benton Test of Facial Recognition (WMS, N = 71; DNS, N = 16), the Warrington Recognition Memory Test (WMS, N = 17; DNS, N = 10), and the Mooney Closure Task (WMS, N = 33; DNS, N = 10), subjects with WMS, despite their marked visuospatial deficits, performed remarkably well; their performance was significantly better

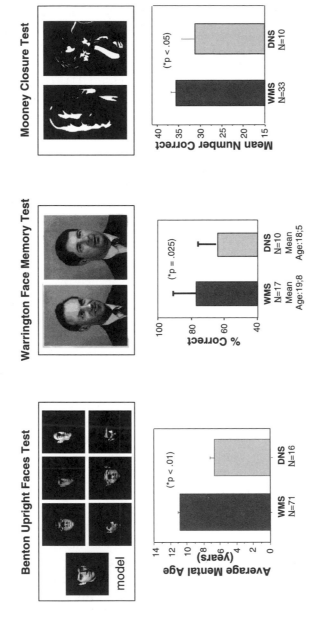

Figure 1.12
Across three tasks involving face processing (Benton Face-Recognition Task, Warrington Face-Memory Task, and Mooney Closure Task), subjects with WMS perform significantly better than their age- and IQ-matched DNS counterparts, indicating that face processing is indeed an area of remarkable sparing in WMS.

than that of subjects with DNS and as proficient as normal age-matched controls (Jones, Rossen, Hickok, Jernigan, & Bellugi, 1995b). Thus, while there are gross deficits in general cognitive abilities, subjects with WMS typically exhibit a distinctive pattern of peaks and valleys in visuo-spatial cognition: An emphasis on local over global processing and extreme fractionation in drawing; yet an island of sparing for processing, recognizing, and remembering faces (Rossen et al., 1995b; Bellugi et al., 1994; Bellugi et al., 1999b).

Dissociation between Spatial Cognition (Impaired) and Face Processing (Spared)   The performance of individuals with WMS on face-processing tasks stands in contrast to their profound impairment on the other visually based cognitive tasks we have described above (drawing, constructing designs of blocks, reproducing hierarchically organized figures). We wondered whether the deficit in WMS might be primarily with tasks that involve spatial construction, or whether the spatial deficit extends to spatial *perception* as well. Two tasks that are nonlinguistic and depend on visual perception only were used to address this question. Both tasks involve processing pictures, and require pointing to the correct answer, but do not involve visuo-constructive abilities. Both tasks were developed by Arthur Benton of the University of Iowa as perceptual tasks that may be especially sensitive to right-hemisphere damage in adults. One is the Judgement of Line Orientation (Benton, Hamsher, Varney, & Spreen, 1983a), a task of spatial cognition that requires a subject to look at a target pair of lines and then point the lines in an array that matches the target pair of lines. The other is the Benton Test of Facial Recognition (Benton et al., 1983b). On the line-orientation task, a sample of 16 subjects with WMS performed in the range considered "severely deficient" for adults; most of those with WMS could not even pass the pretest. In contrast, the group of individuals with WMS who failed the line-orientation task, performed very well, indeed, almost at the normal level for adults, on the face-recognition task (Figure 1.13). In a larger sample of WMS, the same dissociation in visuo-spatial abilities was found: Specifically, subjects with WMS ($N = 23$) performed significantly better on the face-recognition task (mean percent correct = 82.8) than on the task involving line-orientation judgment (mean percent correct = 31.0) ($t = -12.92; p < .0001$).

The Intersection of Space Representation and Language Representation in WMS   As has been discussed thus far, the dissociation between linguistic abilities (disproportionately spared) and visuo-spatial cognitive abilities (disproportionately impaired, except for certain aspects of face processing) is one of the hallmarks of the cognitive profile of WMS. There is a clear spatial-cognitive deficit in nearly all individuals with WMS across both constructive and perceptual realms (observed on tasks that involve copying block designs, drawings, and hierarchical figures, as well as line-orientation

Peaks and Valleys of Ability in Visual Processing in Williams Syndrome: Lines vs. Faces

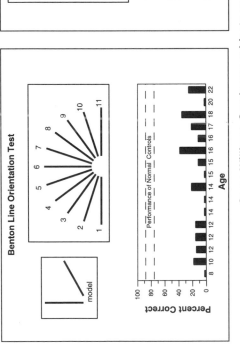

Same Williams Syndrome subjects on contrasting spatial tasks

Figure 1.13

The strengths and weaknesses in visuo-spatial processing in WMS show an unusual profile. The results are shown from two tasks that are both visuo-perceptual tasks, sensitive to right-hemisphere damage, where the correct answer requires only pointing to a picture without any constructional component. Note that the same subjects with WMS perform very differently on the two tasks. The contrast in performance on line orientation (Benton Judgement of Line Orientation, mean percent correct = 92.59) is shown for 16 subjects with WMS ($t = 18.69$; $p < .0001$). On the Line-Orientation task, several individuals with WMS could not even pass the warm up items. In great contrast, exactly the same subjects with WMS perform remarkably well on a very difficult face discrimination task that involves recognizing the same individual under different conditions of lighting, shadow, and orientation. In both tasks, performance of normal individuals is indicated by the broken lines.

judgment) (Bellugi, Lai, & Wang, 1997; Beret, Lai, Hickok, Stiles, & Klima, 1997). In language studies with individuals with WMS, we observe that even adults tend to occasionally misuse spatial prepositions in narratives (Rubba & Klima, 1991). For example, in a story-telling task from a wordless picture book about a boy and his dog and their search for a missing frog, statements are noted such as: "The boy was so sad, his tears were falling off from his eyes"; "The dog has the jar in his face" (the picture shows the dog with his head in a jar). Such errors made by subjects with WMS on this story-telling task suggested that the use of language to describe spatial relations was potentially problematic and warranted further study.

Testing individuals with WMS on tasks that involve the use of both linguistic and spatial abilities may result in different possible outcomes. Their strong language skills may mask their poor spatial abilities, or their poor spatial skills may interfere with their strong language abilities. An investigation of how subjects with WMS use prepositions to describe spatial relations was conducted in order to understand the intersection between their spared language and impaired spatial cognition. Two tasks were developed that measured an individual's ability to comprehend and produce specific spatial prepositions. Data were collected from 28 WMS subjects (mean age: 19; range: 10 to 41 years) and 27 normal controls in the fifth and sixth grade (mean age: 11.25; range: 9.99 to 12.30 years), who were significantly younger than the experimental group (Lichtenberger & Bellugi, 1998).

In a test of comprehension of spatial prepositions, subjects were required to listen to auditorily presented spatial prepositions and choose one of four pictures that best represented the preposition or spatial phrase (e.g., through, between, above, in front of). Despite the age difference between normal control and WMS subjects, normal controls performed significantly better on the spatial preposition comprehension test ($p < .05$). In fact, the normal controls performed at ceiling, making only .2% errors on average. In contrast, the WMS subjects made an average of 11.5% errors.

The second task assessed expressive abilities with spatial language, as tapped by the production of spatial prepositions. In this task, subjects were asked to look at pictures in which a colored item was placed in relation to another item not colored, a task modeled after Bowerman (Bowerman, 1996). For example, a drawing of a boy (colored yellow) was depicted in front of a drawing of a chair, a drawing of an apple (colored yellow) was depicted inside of a transparent bowl. The subject's task was to tell where the shaded item was in relation to the other item. Subjects with WMS again made significantly more errors when compared to the group of younger normally developing subjects ($p < .001$). On average, the WMS group produced errors in 30.2% of their verbal responses, but the group of normally developing children had a significantly smaller

The Dissociation between Language and Spatial Representation in Williams Syndrome

The boy is colored yellow

Target: Boy in front of chair

14 yrs: The boy is yellow and he is standing up right here behind.

18 yrs: The guy s standing beside the chair. His back would be facing.

21 yrs: The boy is standing behind the chair.

The tree is colored yellow

Target: Tree in front of/beside a church

14 years: It s standing on the ground with it s big hairy bouquet high up in the sky.

20 years: Tree behind a church.

21 years: The tree is growing on top of a castle.

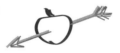

The arrow is colored yellow

Target: Arrow through apple

13 years: Apple is in the bow and arrow.

13 years: The arrow is on an apple.

18 years: An apple with an arrow and the arrow s between the apple and it is inside the apple.

The apple is colored yellow

Target: Apple in bowl

12 years: Apple without the bowl.

13 years: The bowl is in the apple.

13 years: The apple is around the bowl.

Figure 1.14
Experimental tasks were developed to investigate the intersection of language and spatial representation in WMS, including production and comprehension tasks (modeled after Bowerman, 1996). Shown here are sample errors made by WMS individuals ages 12 and older on a task involving production of spatial prepositions and language about space. Note that on the actual stimuli pictures, one of the objects in the picture is colored yellow (but here is shaded) to represent the target item, as in the picture of an arrow passing through an apple. Individuals with WMS exhibit difficulty in the mapping between language and spatial representation, e.g., 'The arrow is on the apple,' or 'An apple with an arrow and the arrow's between the apple and it is inside the apple' (Lichtenberger & Bellugi, 1998).

rate of errors. Examples of the kinds of errors made by the WMS group on the spatial preposition production task are shown in Figure 1.14.

As shown in Figure 1.14, individuals with WMS were noted to make errors in describing the spatial relationships that included *reversing* the subject and object of the sentence and those that were semantically inappropriate in other ways. For the item showing a *tree (colored) in front of (or beside) a church,* none of the normally developing younger children made responses that were irregular other than being atypically general in their descriptions. For example, some of the normally developing subjects responded, "the tree is by the church." However, some of the individuals with WMS made errors such as using a preposition that denotes a spatial relationship opposite from what was pictured, e.g., "tree behind a house," or produced responses that were inappropriate given the target picture, e.g., "the tree is growing on top of a castle." These types of language errors about spatial relationships made by some individuals with WMS in the spatial language production task were never observed even in the younger normally developing group (Lichtenberger & Bellugi, 1998). Thus, from this initial task, it appears that the WMS individuals in particular may be having difficulty in the mapping between spatial representation and language representation. This area of investigation, involving a dissociation between language and spatial representations in WMS, should provide new understanding of the mapping between these domains.

Distinct Developmental Trajectories Across Cognitive Domains

Previous studies have shown that WMS results in a highly uneven profile of specific deficits, preservations, and anomalies both within and across cognitive domains. However, there has been little information available regarding the developmental profile in this rare disorder. A study by Jones, Hickok, Rossen and Bellugi (1998b) (see also Jones, Rossen, & Bellugi, 1995a) examined questions of development of specific cognitive domains in a cross-sectional study of 71 individuals with WMS (ages: 5 to 29 years; mean age: 14.9 years). Using standardized measures of receptive vocabulary, copying drawings, and face recognition, the study examined the patterns of age-related changes in WMS, using individuals with DNS as a basis for comparison.

The results indicate that subjects with WMS perform very differently on the three types of tasks during school-age, adolescence, and adulthood and also show distinct changes across the age range (see Figure 1.15). In the WMS cohort, a specific development trajectory was found for each cognitive domain measured in contrast to the DNS cohort (Figure 1.15). For instance, in the area of receptive vocabulary, children with WMS were found to be significantly delayed early on, but then improved with increasing age. Once past this initial delay in language, subjects with WMS showed an increase in abilities throughout childhood, adolescence, and into adulthood. In contrast,

Distinct Trajectories in Cognitive Domains in Williams Syndrome but not in Down Syndrome

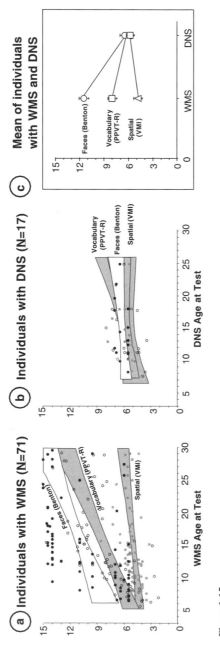

Figure 1.15
Developmental trajectories of contrasts between language, face and space processing in WMS are shown. (a) Subjects of all ages with WMS show distinctly different trajectories in three domains: Lexical knowledge, spatial cognition, and face processing. On a standardized test of vocabulary, subjects with WMS start with low scores and then show a sharp increase with age. On a spatial task that involves copying geometric shapes, the performances of subjects with WMS are consistently below those of subjects with DNS, and plateau at an early age. On a task of face processing, subjects with WMS perform extremely well even at very young ages. (b) Subjects with DNS showed essentially the same developmental trajectory across the three domains. In contrast, subjects with WMS show three distinctly different trajectories. (c) Planned contrasts show that performance on the three tests differs significantly within the WMS group, even when controlled for age. No between-test differences are found in the DNS group (reproduced from Jones et al., 1998a; Jones et al., 1998b).

in the visuospatial domain, subjects with WMS showed pronounced impairment and limited change in ability across the age-range studied. Development of face-recognition abilities in WMS was distinct from development in the visuospatial and receptive vocabulary abilities in the study. With face recognition, young children with WMS performed at a higher level, on average, than would be expected for their age, and performed well throughout development. In contrast to the other areas sampled, the face recognition can be characterized as a relative strength for WMS across the age span.

The WMS findings are even more impressive when they are compared to an age-matched sample of individuals with DNS (ages: 7 to 28 years; mean age: 14.5 years). The DNS group performed similarly on all three standardized tasks of receptive vocabulary, spatial ability and face processing (see Figure 1.15). Thus, there was no evidence of age-related changes in DNS in the separate cognitive domains involved. In contrast, three distinctly different trajectories of development across age were found in WMS, yielding evidence for the separability of language, spatial abilities, and face processing in human behavior. Subjects with WMS present a rare opportunity to study the separability of cognitive domains that normally develop together, and to characterize the trajectories of their development across the age span (Bellugi et al., 1999b).

Cognitive Domains in Williams Syndrome Subjects

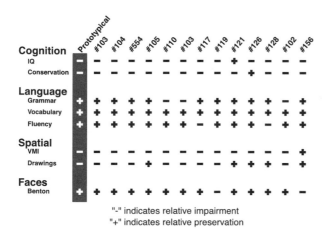

"-" indicates relative impairment
"+" indicates relative preservation

Figure 1.16
The prototypical cognitive phenotype for individuals with WMS is shown for the domains of cognition, language, spatial ability, and face processing ability. Most of the individuals in this WMS sample have cognitive profiles that show similar areas of relative impairment and relative strength.

Consistency (and Variability) in the Williams Cognitive Phenotype The studies discussed in this paper, as well as in the other papers that follow in this volume, provide the opportunity to link variability in the phenotypic expression of the cognitive profile to variability in the expression of markers of brain structure, brain function and, ultimately, the gene. We have focused on the prototypical cognitive profile of WMS, which appears to distinguish this syndrome from DNS and, perhaps, other syndromes as well (see also Mervis et al., 1999). At the same time, we can address the extent to which there is some variability within the consistent profile of dissociations in higher cognitive function in WMS. Figure 1.16 shows aspects of the prototypical profile of WMS showing peaks and valleys of abilities within cognitive functions which we have so far elucidated—impairment in general cognition as measured by IQ tests, disproportionate strength in aspects of language, co-occurring with marked spatial cognitive deficits but excellent face processing. In addition to scores from such general cognition batteries as the WISC-R and WAIS-R, we now have a large database of results from general cognitive, language, and visuo-spatial tasks on a significant number of individuals with WMS. We are quantifying what is typical, or the "normal-range" of functioning, for WMS on each of the standardized tests in our database. Thus, we can examine the extent to which each individual diagnosed with WMS falls within or outside the range of what is typical (or "normal" for WMS) as a group. Studies of the variability in neurobehavioral profile within WMS are proving critical for exposing the relationships between cognitive and neural phenotypes and, ultimately, the genotype.

Social, Neural, and Genetic Markers: Elucidating the Phenotype In this broad program studying the phenotype of WMS, we have described the cognitive profile and are now in a position to expand the phenotypic description to include social, neural, and genetic aspects of WMS. Studies of WMS social behavior described in the next chapter show that the behavioral phenotype also typically includes a type of "hypersociability." WMS individuals tend to be overly friendly with strangers, and even as infants show more positive and less negative behavior than normals in social situations, and are dramatic story tellers (Jones et al., chap. 2; Bellugi et al., 1998). This highly social interpersonal style noted in formal testing as well as in experimental paradigms provides another critical (and quantifiable) aspect of the WMS phenotype, marking it as different from normal and directly opposite from autism.

Our studies of brain function and brain morphology suggest that there are neural abnormalities that also serve as markers for WMS, distinguishing aspects of the neurobiological phenotype (Bellugi et al., 1999a). There are unique electrophysiological patterns present during paradigms of language processing and face processing (Mills et al., 1997; Mills, 1998; Mills et al., chap. 3). These distinctive electrophysiological patterns which are characteristic of WMS are different from those found with normal controls at any age or from other groups. Additional neural characteristics providing possible markers of WMS

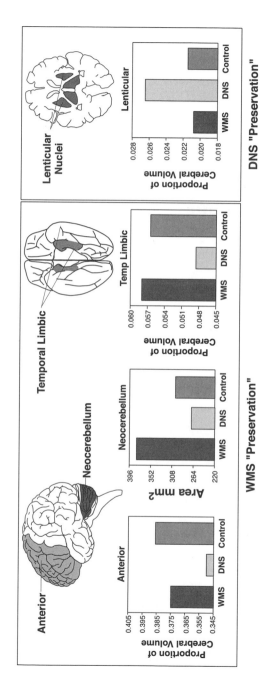

Figure 1.17
In vivo MRI studies involving computer-graphic analysis of brains of individuals with WMS suggest an anomalous morphological profile that consists of a distinct regional pattern of proportional brain volume deficits and preservations. (a) There is relative preservation of anterior-cortical areas and enlargement of neo-cerebellar areas in WMS subjects. These are two areas that have undergone the most prominent enlargement in the human brain relative to lower primates. (b) There is relative preservation of mesial-temporal lobe in WMS subjects. In conjunction with certain areas of frontal cortex, this area is thought to mediate certain aspects of affective functioning. (c) In DNS individuals, there is relative preservation of subcortical areas (lenticular nuclei) that is not seen in WMS, perhaps relevant to the significantly better motor skills in DNS subjects (adapted from Bellugi et al., 1996b).

Gene Deletion in Williams Syndrome

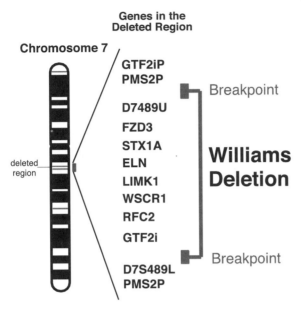

**Genes in the
Deleted Region**

Chromosome 7

GTF2iP
PMS2P

Breakpoint

D7489U

FZD3

STX1A

ELN

LIMK1

WSCR1

RFC2

GTF2i

**Williams
Deletion**

deleted
region

Breakpoint

D7S489L
PMS2P

Figure 1.18
A genetic marker for WMS is the deletion of one copy of a small set of genes on chromosome 7, band 7q1l23, shown in the ideogram. This region is expanded to the right to illustrate genes that are missing one copy in WMS, including the gene for elastin. The regions involving the common breakpoints in WMS are also illustrated (see Korenberg et al., chap. 6). Thus, WMS is characterized genetically by deletion of one copy of a small set of genes on chromosome 7, including the gene for elastin (illustration based on Korenberg et al., 1998).

include enlargement of the neocerebellar vermis in the context of an overall smaller brain size (see Figure 1.17), and differential development of the paleocerebellum (small) and the neocerebellum (enlarged) in WMS (Jernigan & Bellugi, 1994; Bellugi et al., 1994; Bellugi & Wang, 1998) as well as disordered neurons on histology (Galaburda, Wang, Bellugi, & Rossen, 1994; Galaburda, 1998; Galaburda & Bellugi, chap. 5).

Beyond these neural characteristics, the deletion of one copy of a small set of genes in a distinct region on chromosome 7 (band 7q11.23) characterizes nearly all clinically identified WMS and provides a genetic marker for WMS (Bellugi et al., 1999b; Korenberg et al., 1996, Korenberg et al., 1997, Korenberg et al., 1998; Korenberg et al., chap. 6). Figure 1.18 shows a simplified diagram of the hemizygous deletion in a small region on chromosome 7, and some of the genes in that region that are currently being identified (see Korenberg et al., chap. 6).

The cognitive profile of Williams syndrome represents an unusual pattern of strengths and weaknesses, indeed, dissociations within and across cognitive domains, as we have shown in this chapter. Phenotypic characteristics of WMS at the social, neural, and genetic levels, provide an additional opportunity to forge links from cognition to underlying neural substrates and to the genetic basis of the syndrome.

Conclusion

The results of these studies should provide clues to long-standing theoretical issues in language and brain organization and, in addition, have the potential for connecting the cognitive and social profile of a specific genetically based disorder, with its brain bases, and with its genetic underpinnings. We are investigating major dissociations among and within diverse cognitive functions: Selectively spared grammatical capacity in the face of marked cognitive deficits. Dissociations within language (grammar, semantics) as well as within other domains of cognition (impaired spatial cognition, remarkably spared face processing) are also present. In subsequent papers, we explore these dissociations in terms of their implications for the neural systems underlying cognitive domains and their implications for neuronal plasticity. One of the greatest challenges in understanding the brain basis of higher cortical functions lies in being able to link investigations across disciplines within the neurosciences.

Notes

This research was supported by grants to Ursula Bellugi at the Salk Institute from the National Institutes of Health (P01 HD33113, P50 NS22343, PO1 DC01289), the OakTree Philanthropic Foundation, and the James S. McDonnell Foundation. The authors thank the National and Regional Williams Syndrome Associations and the National and Regional Down Syndrome Associations. The authors are grateful to Edward S. Klima for his helpful comments. The authors would like to thank the subjects and their families for their spirited participation in these studies.

Illustrations and quotes not to be used without written permission from the author. Copyright Dr. Ursula Bellugi, La Jolla, CA.

References

Atkinson, J., King, J., Braddick, O., & Nokes, L. (1997). A specific deficit of dorsal stream function in Williams syndrome. *NeuroReport, 8,* 1919–1922.

Bates, E. (1997). On language savants and the structure of the mind: A review of Neil Smith and Ianthi-Maria Tsimpli, "The mind of a savant: Language learning and modularity." *International Journal of Bilingualism, 1,* 163–179.

Beery, K. E. (1997). *The Beery-Buktenica developmental test of visual-motor integration* (4th ed., Revised). Parsippany, NJ: Modern Curriculum Press.

Bellugi, U. (1998). Symposium, bridging cognition, brain and gene: Evidence from Williams syndrome. Abstract, *Cognitive Neuroscience Society 1998 Annual Meeting Abstract Program*, 9–11.

Bellugi, U., Bihrle, A., Jernigan, T., Trauner, D., & Doherty, S. (1990). Neuropsychological, neurological, and neuroanatomical profile of Williams syndrome. *American Journal of Medical Genetics, 6*, 115–125.

Bellugi, U., Bihrle, A., Neville H., Jernigan, T., & Doherty, S. (1992). Language, cognition and brain organization in a neurodevelopmental disorder. In M. Gunnar & C. Nelson (Eds.), *Developmental behavioral neuroscience* (pp. 201–232). Hillsdale, NJ: Erlbaum.

Bellugi, U., Hickok, G., Jones, W., & Jernigan, T. (1996a). The neurobiological basis of Williams syndrome: Linking brain and behavior. *Williams Syndrome Association Professional Conference*, King of Prussia, PA.

Bellugi, U., Klima, E. S., & Wang, P. P. (1996b). Cognitive and neural development: Clues from genetically based syndromes. In D. Magnussen (Ed.), *The life-span development of individuals: Behavioral, neurobiological, and psychosocial perspectives* (pp. 223–243). The Nobel Symposium. New York, NY: Cambridge University Press.

Bellugi, U., Lai, Z., & Wang, P. P. (1997). Language, communication, and neural systems in Williams syndrome. *Mental Retardation and Developmental Disabilities Research Review, 3*, 334–342.

Bellugi, U., Lichtenberger, L., Mills, D., Galaburda, A., & Korenberg, J. (1999a). Bridging cognition, brain and molecular genetics: Evidence from Williams syndrome. *Trends in Neurosciences, 22*, 197–207.

Bellugi, U., Losh, M., Reilly, J., & Anderson, D. (1998). *Excessive use of linguistically encoded affect: Stories from young children with Williams syndrome* (Technical Report CND-9801). University of California, San Diego, Center for Research in Language, Project in Cognitive and Neural Development.

Bellugi, U., Mills, D., Jernigan, T., Hickok, G., & Galaburda, A. (1999b). Linking cognition, brain structure and brain function in Williams syndrome. In H. Tager-Flusberg (Ed.), *Neurodevelopmental disorders: Contributions to a new framework from the cognitive neurosciences* (pp. 111–136). Cambridge, MA: MIT Press.

Bellugi, U., & Morris, C. (Eds.) (1995). Williams syndrome: From cognition to gene. In J. P. Fryns (Ed.), *Abstracts from the Williams Syndrome Association Professional Conference* [Special Issue]. *Genetic counseling, 6*, 131–192.

Bellugi, U., & Wang, P. P. (1998). Williams syndrome: From cognition to brain to gene. In G. Edelman & B. H. Smith (Eds.), *Encyclopedia of neuroscience*. Amsterdam, the Netherlands: Elsevier; CD-ROM version, New York, NY: Elsevier.

Bellugi, U., Wang, P. P., & Jernigan, T. L. (1994). Williams syndrome: An unusual neuropsychological profile. In S. Broman & J. Grafman (Eds.), *Atypical cognitive deficits in developmental disorders: Implications for brain function* (pp. 23–56). Hillsdale, NJ: Erlbaum.

Benton, A. L., Hamsher, K. de S., Varney, N. R., & Spreen, O. (1983a). *Benton judgment of line orientation, form H.* New York, NY: Oxford University Press.

Benton, A. L., Hamsher, K. de S., Varney, N. R., & Spreen, O. (1983b). *Benton test of facial recognition.* New York, NY: Oxford University Press.

Beret, N., Bellugi, U., Hickok, G., & Stiles, J. (1996, July). Integrative spatial deficits in children with Williams syndrome and children with focal brain lesions: A comparison. *Williams Syndrome Association Professional Conference*, King of Prussia, PA.

Beret, N., Lai, Z. C., Hickok, G., Stiles, J., & Klima, E. S. (1997). Spatial integrative deficits in Williams syndrome: Comparison with right hemisphere damage. *International Behavioral Neuroscience Society Abstracts, 6*, 58, P2–47.

Bihrle, A. M. (1990). *Visuospatial processing in Williams and Down syndrome.* Unpublished Doctoral Dissertation, University of California at San Diego and San Diego State University. (Abstracted 1991 in *Dissertation Abstracts International, 52* (2-B), 1048.)

Bihrle, A. M., Bellugi, U., Delis, D., & Marks, S. (1989). Seeing either the forest or the trees: Dissociation in visuospatial processing. *Brain and Cognition, 11*, 37–49.

Bishop, D. M. (1982). *Test for reception of grammar.* Abingdon, England: Thomas Leach.

Bowerman, M. (1996). Learning how to structure space for language: A crosslinguistic perspective. In P. Bloom & M. A. Peterson, et al. (Eds.), *Language and space* (pp. 385–436). Cambridge, MA: MIT Press.

Carey, S. (1985). *Conceptual change in childhood.* Cambridge, MA: MIT Press.

Carrow, E. (1974). *Carrow elicited language inventory.* Boston, MA: Teaching Resources.

Clahsen, H., & Almazan, M. (1998). Syntax and morphology in Williams syndrome. *Cognition, 68,* 167–198.

Curtiss, S., & Yamada, J. (1988). *The Curtiss-Yamada comprehensive language evaluation (CYCLE).* Unpublished test. University of California, Los Angeles, CA.

Dehaene, S. (1997). *The number sense: How the mind creates mathematics.* New York: Oxford University Press.

Dennis, M., & Whitaker, H. A. (1976). Language acquisition following hemidecortication: Linguistic superiority of the left over the right hemisphere. *Brain and Language, 3,* 404–433.

Dunn, L. M., & Dunn, L. M. (1981). *Peabody picture vocabulary tests—revised manual.* Circle Pines, MN: American Guidance Service.

Einfeld, S. L. Tonge, B. J., & Florio, T. (1997). Behavioral and emotional disturbance in individuals with Williams syndrome. *American Journal of Psychiatry, 102,* 45–53.

Fenson, L., Dale, P., Reznick, S., Thal, D., Bates, E., Hartung, J., Pethick, S., & Reilly, J. (1993). *MacArthur communicative development inventories: Technical manual.* San Diego, CA: Singular Publishing Group.

Frangiskakis, J. M., Ewart, A. K., Morris, C. A., Mervis, C. B., Bertrand, J., Robinson, B. F., Klein, B. P., Ensing, G. J., Everett, L. A., Green, E. D., Proschel, C., Gutowski, N. J., Noble, M., Atkinson, D. L., Odelberg, S. J., & Keating, M. T. (1996). LIM-kinase hemizygosity implicated in impaired visuospatial constructive cognition. *Cell, 86,* 59–69.

Galaburda, A. M. (1998). Brain cytoarchitectonic findings in Williams syndrome. *Cognitive Neuroscience Society 1998 Annual Meeting Abstract Program, 10*–11.

Galaburda, A., & Bellugi, U. (chap. 5). Cellular and molecular cortical neuroanatomy in Williams syndrome.

Galaburda, A., Wang, P. P., Bellugi, U., & Rossen, M. L. (1994). Cytoarchitectonic findings in a genetically based disorder: Williams syndrome. *NeuroReport, 5,* 758–787.

Howlin, P., Davies, M., & Udwin, O. (1998). Cognitive functioning in adults with Williams syndrome. *Journal of Child Psychology and Psychiatry, 39,* 183–189.

Jernigan, T. L., & Bellugi, U. (1994). Neuroanatomical distinctions between Williams and Down syndromes. In S. Broman & J. Grafman (Eds.), *Atypical cognitive deficits in developmental disorders: Implications in brain function* (pp. 57–66). Hillsdale, NJ: Erlbaum.

Johnson, S. C., & Carey, S. (1998). Knowledge enrichment and conceptual change in folkbiology: Evidence from Williams syndrome. *Cognitive Psychology, 37,* 156–200.

Jones, W., Bellugi, U., Lai, Z., Chiles, M., Reilly, J., Lincoln, A., & Adolphs, R. (chap. 2). Hypersociability: The social and affective phenotype of Williams syndrome.

Jones, W., Hickok, G., & Lai, Z. (1998a). Does face processing rely on intact visual-spatial abilities? Evidence from Williams Syndrome. *Cognitive Neuroscience Society Abstract program, 80*(67).

Jones, W., Hickok, G., Rossen, M. L., & Bellugi, U. (1998b). *Dissociations in cognitive development: Differential effects from two genetically based syndromes* (Tech. Rep. No. CND-9805). San Diego, CA: University of California, Center for Research in Language, Project in Cognitive and Neural Development.

Jones, W., Rossen, M. L., & Bellugi, U. (1995a). Distinct developmental trajectories of cognition in Williams syndrome. Abstract, Special Issue, *Genetic Counseling, 6,* 178–179.

Jones, W., Rossen, M. L., Hickok, G., Jernigan, T., & Bellugi, U. (1995b). Links between behavior and brain: Brain morphological correlates of language, face, and auditory processing in Williams syndrome. *Society for Neuroscience Abstracts, 21,* 1926.

Karmiloff-Smith, A. (1998). Development itself is the key to understanding developmental disorders. *Trends in Cognitive Sciences, 2,* 289–298.

Karmiloff-Smith, A., Grant, J., Berthoud, J., Davies, M., Howlin, P., & Udwin, O. (1997). Language in Williams syndrome: How intact is 'intact?' *Child Development, 68,* 246–262.

Kempler, D., & VanLanker, D. (1993). Sentence comprehension in Parkinson's disease. *ASHA Abstracts, 35,* 176.

Kopera-Frye, K., Dehaene, S., & Streissguth, A. P. (1996). Impairments of number processing induced by prenatal alcohol exposure. *Neuropsychologia, 34,* 1187–1196.

Korenberg, J., Chen, X.-N., Hirota, H., Lai, Z., Bellugi, U., Burian, D., Roe, B., & Matsuoka, R. (chap. 6). Genome structure and cognitive map of Williams Syndrome.

Korenberg, J. R., Chen, X.-N., Lai, Z., Yimlamai, D., Bishighini, R., & Bellugi, U. (1997). Williams syndrome. The search for genetic origins of cognition. *American Journal of Human Genetics, 61,* A103, 579.

Korenberg, J. R., Chen, X.-N., Mitchell, S., Sun, Z.-G., Hubert, R., Vataru, E. S., & Bellugi, U. (1996). The genomic organization of Williams syndrome. *American Journal of Medical Genetics Supplement, 59,* A306, 1776.

Korenberg, J. R., Hirota, H., Chen, X-N., Lai, Z., Yimlamai, D., Matsuoka, R., & Bellugi, U. (1998). The molecular genetic basis of Williams syndrome. *Cognitive Neuroscience Society 1998 Annual Meeting Abstract Program,* 10.

Lenhoff, H. M., Wang, P. P., Greenberg, F., & Bellugi, U. (1997). Williams syndrome and the brain. *Scientific American, 277,* 68–73.

Levy, Y. (1996). Modularity of language reconsidered. *Brain and Language, 55,* 240–263.

Lichtenberger, L., & Bellugi, U. (1998). The intersection of spatial cognition and language in Williams syndrome. Abstract, *Cognitive Neuroscience Society 1998 Annual Meeting Abstract Program, 80*(68).

Marriage, J., & Scientist, A. (1995). Central auditory hyperacusis in Williams syndrome. In U. Bellugi & C. A. Morris (Eds.), Williams syndrome: From cognition to gene. Abstracts from the Williams Syndrome Association Professional Conference. Special Issue, *Genetic Counseling, 6,* 131–192.

Mervis, C. B., Morris, C. A., Bertrand, J., & Robinson, B. F. (1999). Williams syndrome: Findings from an integrated program of research. In H. Tager-Flusberg (Ed.), *Neurodevelopmental disorders: Contributions to a new framework from the cognitive neurosciences* (pp. 65–110). Cambridge, MA: MIT Press.

Mills, D. L. (1998). Electrophysiological markers for Williams syndrome. *Cognitive Neuroscience Society 1998 Annual Meeting Abstract Program,* 10.

Mills, D., Alvarez, T., St. George, Appelbaum, L. M., Bellugi, U., & Neville, H. (chap. 3). Neurophysiological markers of face processing in Williams Syndrome.

Mills, D., Neville, H., Appelbaum, G., Prat, C., & Bellugi, U. (1997). Electrophysiological markers of Williams syndrome. *International Behavioral Neuroscience Society Abstracts, 6*(P2-50), 59.

Mooney, C. M. (1957). Age in the development of closure ability in children. *Canadian Journal of Psychology, 11,* 219–226.

Pinker, S. (1994). *The language instinct.* New York, NY: Harper Perennial.

Pinker, S. (1997). Words and rules in the human brain. *Nature, 387,* 547–548.

Reiss, A., Eliez, S., Schmitt, J. E., Straus, E., Lai, Z., Jones, W., & Bellugi, U. (chap. 4). Neuroanatomy of Williams syndrome: A high-resolution MRI study.

Reitan, R., & Wolfson, D. (1985). *The Halstead-Reitan neuropsychological test battery: Theory and clinical interpretation.* Tucson, AZ: Neuropsychology Press.

Rossen, M. L., Jones, W., Wang, P. P., & Klima, E. S. (1995a). Face processing: Remarkable sparing in Williams syndrome. Special Issue, *Genetic Counseling, 6,* 138–140.

Rossen, M. L., Klima, E. S., Bellugi, U., Bihrle, A., & Jones, W. (1996). Interaction between language and cognition: Evidence from Williams syndrome. In J. H. Beitchman, N. Cohen, M. Konstantareas, & R. Tannock (Eds.), *Language, learning, and behavior disorders: Developmental, biological, and clinical perspectives* (pp. 367–392). New York, NY: Cambridge University Press.

Rossen, M. L., Smith, D., Jones, W., Bellugi, U., & Korenberg, J. R. (1995b). Spared face processing in Williams syndrome: New perspectives on brain-behavior links in a genetically-based syndrome. *Society for Neuroscience Abstracts, 21,* 1926.

Rubba, J., & Klima, E. S. (1991). Preposition use in a speaker with Williams syndrome: Some cognitive grammar proposals. *Center for Research on Language Newsletter, University of California, La Jolla, CA, 5,* 3–12.

Semel, E., Wiig, E. H., & Secord, W. (1987). *Clinical evaluation of language fundamentals—revised (CELF-R).* San Antonio, TX: The Psychological Corporation.

Singer-Harris, N. G., Bellugi, U., Bates, E., Jones, W., & Rossen, M. L. (1997). Contrasting profiles of language development in children with Williams and Down syndromes. In D. J. Thal & J. S. Reilly (Eds.), Special Issue: "Origins of Language Disorders," *Developmental Neuropsychology, 13,* 345–370.

Stevens, T., & Karmiloff-Smith, A. (1997). Word learning in a special population: Do individuals with Williams syndrome obey lexical constraints? *Journal of Child Language, 24,* 737–765.

Stiles-Davis, J., Kritchevsky, M., & Bellugi, U. (1988). *Spatial cognition: Brain bases and development.* Hillsdale, NJ: Erlbaum.

Udwin, O. (1990). A survey of adults with Williams syndrome and idiopathic infantile hypercalcaemia. *Developmental Medicine and Child Neurology, 32,* 129–141.

Volterra, V., Capirci, O., Pezzini, G., Sabbadini, L., & Vicari, S. (1996). Linguistic abilities in Italian children with Williams syndrome. *Cortex, 32,* 663–677.

Wang, P. P., & Bellugi, U. (1993). Williams syndrome, Down syndrome and cognitive neuroscience. *American Journal of Diseases of Children, 147,* 1246–1251.

Wang, P. P., Doherty, S., Rourke, S. B., & Bellugi, U. (1995). Unique profile of visuo-perceptual skills in a genetic syndrome. *Brain and Cognition, 29,* 54–65.

Warrington, E. K. (1984). *Warrington recognition memory test.* Windsor, England: Nfer-Nelson Publishing.

Wechsler, D. (1974). *Wechsler intelligence scale for children—revised.* San Antonio, TX: The Psychological Corporation.

Wechsler, D. (1981). *Wechsler adult intelligence scale—revised.* San Antonio, TX: The Psychological Corporation.

2 Hypersociability: The Social and Affective Phenotype of Williams Syndrome

Wendy Jones, Ursula Bellugi, Zona Lai, Michael Chiles, Judy Reilly, Alan Lincoln, and Ralph Adolphs

Studies of abnormal populations provide a rare opportunity for examining relationships between cognition, genotype and brain neurobiology, permitting comparisons across these different levels of analysis. In our studies, we investigate individuals with a rare, genetically based disorder called Williams syndrome (WMS) to draw links among these levels. A critical component of such a cross-domain undertaking is the clear delineation of the phenotype of the disorder in question. Of special interest in this is a relatively unexplored unusual social phenotype in WMS that includes an overfriendly and engaging personality. Four studies measuring distinct aspects of hypersocial behavior in WMS are presented, each probing specific aspects in WMS infants, toddlers, school age children, and adults. The abnormal profile of excessively social behavior represents an important component of the phenotype that may distinguish WMS from other developmental disorders. Furthermore, the studies show that the profile is observed across a wide range of ages, and emerges consistently across multiple experimental paradigms. These studies of hypersocial behavior in WMS promise to provide the groundwork for crossdisciplinary analyses of gene-brain-behavior relationships.

Introduction

One of the great challenges in understanding the genetic and brain bases of behaviors is to link studies across different levels of investigation. Studies of syndromes that involve atypical cognition, brain organization, and molecular genetic structure provide an opportunity to link such domains. There has been considerable progress in cross-domain studies in the neurosciences, especially in the cognitive neurosciences, over the past decade using Williams syndrome (WMS) as a model (Bellugi, Lichtenberger, Mills, Galaburda, & Korenberg, 1999b; Bellugi, Mills, Jernigan, Hickok, & Galaburda, 1999c; and chapters in this volume). Advances in techniques across disciplines have improved cross-domain research, leading to a better understanding of the neural bases of mental capacities, such as language, spatial abilities, face processing, and human social behavior.

The aim of the current set of studies is to investigate the neural and genetic bases of social behavior in WMS, a genetic disorder of particular interest due to pronounced abnormalities in the social domain. The paper integrates information from several sources to define a social phenotype for WMS. Individuals with WMS are contrasted with individuals who have other genetically based syndromes, such as Down syndrome (DNS) and Autism, as well as with normal control subjects, to understand which particular aspects of abnormal social behavior are specific to WMS, and to examine the relationships between social behavior and other aspects of cognition in WMS. The findings suggest that a strong drive toward social interaction makes up an important and distinctive part of the WMS behavioral phenotype. In addition, we suggest that the specification of a social profile in WMS may provide the means for cross-level analyses of the neuroanatomical, neurophysiological and genetic bases of the disorder.

What Is Williams Syndrome?

WMS is a rare, genetically based disorder caused by the absence of one copy of approximately 20 genes on chromosome 7, including the genes for elastin, syntaxin 1A, Frizzled, and Lim1kinase, among others (Korenberg et al, chap. 6; Korenberg et al., 1996; Ewart et al., 1993). The genetic deletion typically results in mild to moderate mental retardation evidenced from standardized tests of intelligence, but a fractionated cognitive profile. Indeed, WMS individuals have poor spatial skills, but are relatively good at certain other cognitive abilities, including language production and the processing of faces (Bellugi et al., chap. 1; Jones, Hickok, Rossen, & Bellugi, 1999a; Mervis, Morris, Bertrand, & Robinson, 1999; Rossen, Klima, Bellugi, Bihrle, & Jones, 1996). The dissociations seen in the WMS cognitive profile are of particular interest to researchers because they offer an opportunity to identify subcomponents that are dissociable in cognition. In most studies of WMS, individuals with WMS are matched to those with other syndromes (e.g., DNS and Autism) on age and/or IQ; the differences between WMS and other disorders are then examined using probes that are domain-specific (see Bellugi et al., chap. 1).

Why Studies of WMS Contribute to Understanding Sociability

Results from several studies suggest that there is also a characteristic personality and social nature in WMS individuals, although the facets of this personality profile are still being defined. Studies show that people with WMS display extensive anxiety and have behavioral problems, as do individuals with other disorders that result in mental retardation (VanLieshout, DeMeyer, Curfs, & Fryns, 1998; Einfeld, Tonge, & Florio, 1997). However, there has been a growing body of evidence (from clinical and laboratory studies, parental report, and from our own observations of several hundred subjects) that WMS individuals may be unusually sociable, friendly, and empathic (see reports in this article and Tager-Flusberg, Sullivan, Boshart, Guttman, & Levine, 1996). For instance, in circumstances typically eliciting social reservation (e.g., encountering strangers), infants, toddlers, children, and adults with WMS frequently come directly up to and begin engaging strangers. Parents report attempts to train their WMS child (e.g., adolescent daughter) *not* to talk to strangers—to no avail. The parent may then watch in private horror as their WMS daughter walks up to a complete stranger in a public place, looks him right in the eye and then asks in a friendly and engaging manner, "Are you a stranger?" Other WMS children and adults in our experience announce that there is no such thing as a stranger; they say (and behave as if) everyone in the world is their friend. Quantifiable measurement in this domain of unrestrained social behavior toward strangers can make a contribution to understanding the unusual phenotype of WMS. Moreover, these studies are relevant to ongoing and future cross-domain research examining "hypersociability" relative to the anatomical and genetic bases of the disorder.

Background to Studies

The results reported in this chapter are part of a coordinated program aimed at characterizing the cognitive, social and genetic profile of WMS. The paper is divided into four sections, each section containing one or more studies. Section I examines the intersection between social expression and language in WMS. It uses results from narrative, storytelling and biographical interview tasks to investigate clues to the WMS social profile through language, examining the intersection of affect and language. This represents the work carried out by J. Reilly, U. Bellugi, M. Losh, and E. Klima. Section II explores the origins of sociability and affect in infants and toddlers with WMS. Studies in this section make use of an experimental paradigm to measure emotional expression in structured situations, such as parental separation. These studies were carried out by W. Jones and J. Reilly. In Section III, the issue of indiscriminate sociability and overfriendliness (i.e., the overwhelming predilection to seek out and engage in conversation with strangers) in adolescents and adults is examined, using an experimental task designed to measure approachability and interest in unfamiliar people. This section represents studies carried out by U. Bellugi, R. Adolphs, and associates. Section IV investigates parental report of social behavior in three contrasting groups: WMS, DNS, and Autistic subjects. It brings out the contrasts between the withdrawn asocial behavior of autistic individuals and the hypersociability of WMS individuals. This section represents studies carried out by U. Bellugi, A. Lincoln, Z. Lai, M. Chiles, and W. Jones. Taken together, the series of studies reported in the chapter highlight, for the first time, the hypersociability of individuals with WMS as an important and quantifiable aspect of the WMS behavioral phenotype.

Subject Selection for Studies

The WMS participants in the studies reported were required to have been diagnosed by a medical geneticist or dysmorphologist familiar with WMS. In addition, each subject met criteria for the syndrome according to the WMS Diagnostic Scoresheet developed by the Williams Syndrome Medical Advisory Board (see also for clinical definitions Morris, Demsey, Leonard, Dilts, & Blackburn, 1988; Preus, 1984). The diagnosis of WMS was genetically confirmed when possible, using markers for deletion of one copy of the elastin gene on chromosome 7 (Korenberg et al., chap. 6). DNS subjects, when included as a basis of comparison for the effects of mild to moderate mental retardation (Studies I and IV), had been diagnosed with trisomy 21, a genetic marker for a form of DNS. Subjects with autism included in Study IV, recruited by A. Lincoln from his autism studies, were included if they met DSM-IV criteria for autism and also achieved scores in the moderate-to-severe autistic range on the Childhood Autism Rating Scale (CARS; Schopler, Reichler, DeVellis, & Daly, 1980). Normal control subjects were included only if there was no evidence of neurological or medical abnormality, or of developmental delay. Subjects from all groups were screened and excluded from the studies if there was evidence of visual, auditory or neurological abnormalities more severe than typically seen in each population.

Results

Section I. Linguistic Expression as an Index of Sociability in WMS

Section I presents the results of studies comparing children and adolescents with WMS to age-matched adolescents with DNS, as well as to normal controls. The interaction between affect and language is explored through the use of interviews and storytelling tasks. The studies investigate the use of social engagement devices in linguistic expression, within the highly structured context of a pictorially guided story, as well as in the more informal context of a "warm-up" interview. The results indicate that people with WMS make extensive, and even excessive, use of expressive linguistic devices to engage and involve their audience in both narrative and interview situations. The use of such expressive linguistic devices to engage an audience provides the first index of the WMS hypersocial nature and drive.

Interviews and storytelling tasks provide a perfect context to investigate linguistic and affective expression. Linguistically, an individual must convey information about the characters and events of the story in a logical and temporally coherent manner. By recruiting the appropriate grammatical devices, the sequence of events and their temporal relations can be made clear, representing the plot of the story. Cognitively, one must make many types of inferences concerning motivation for actions or behaviors of the various characters and the logical connections between events. These elements reflect the narrator's assessment of the meaning or significance of the events of the story (cognitive evaluation), and might be considered to convey one aspect of evaluative function as identified by Labov and Waletsky (1967). In addition, telling a story is a social activity, and an important type of evaluation concerns the relationship of the narrator to the audience. Such elements have been termed social evaluation, and they serve to elicit and maintain the listener's attention (Reilly, Klima, & Bellugi, 1990). Narratives, thus, permit us to address questions regarding the relationship of language to both cognitive and social evaluative propensities.

Short verbal descriptions of pictures provided the first clue that aspects of linguistic expression are abnormally infused with linguistic evaluations, emotional expression, and audience engagement devices in WMS. For instance, Figure 2.1 shows the

Description of Cookie Theft Picture

Examiner: I want you to look at the picture and tell me everything that is going on.

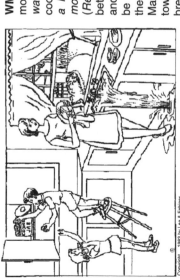

WMS Age 10: (*Laughs*). Oh no. The mommy left the tap on (*pointing to the water*). And the boy is trying to get a cookie but the chair is tipping over. (*In a high voice, as if addressed to the mother*) Mom, won't you save the boy? (*Returning to normal tone*) Gosh. She better quickly save her boy. Her son and her daughter. Oh, there's going to be a flood on her floor. The boy's in the cookies. Maybe it's after supper. Maybe. Oh, the mommy is drying the towel. Poor boy, he could get hurt and break his arm. Poor boy, oh poor thing.

DNS Age 10: Mom wash dishes. A bowl fell. Boy slips, boy pushed. Boy helps mom with dishes. Mom big mess in water. Pushing. (Examiner: Can you tell me anything else about the picture?) (*shakes head*.)

© Copyright 1983 by Lea & Febiger

Figure 2.1
Individuals with WMS tell stories that are not only longer and more complex than those told by same-age subjects with DNS, their narratives are infused with expressive details as well.

responses of a child with WMS and a child with DNS when asked to describe a complex picture. The WMS narrative is longer and more linguistically complex than the DNS narrative and, importantly for this section, contains numerous instances of exaggerated affective expression (e.g., "Poor boy, he could get hurt and break his arm. Poor boy, oh poor thing.").

An initial study on a small group of WMS adolescents followed up on this observation using a storytelling task (Reilly et al., 1990). Participants were asked to construct a narrative on the basis of a series of pictures from a storybook. The narratives were coded for the storyteller's use of lexical evaluative devices including: (a) social devices, such as character speech, sound effects, and affective states; (b) cognitive devices, such as inferences, causal connectors, mental states; and (c) vocal prosody, such as the use of vocal pitch changes, vocal lengthening, and changes in vocal volume. See Bamburg and Reilly (1996) for additional methods used in analyzing narratives in developmental populations.

Results from the first narrative study showed that adolescents and adults with WMS constructed coherent and complex stories that made use of high levels of lexical evaluative devices and vocal prosody (see Figure 2.2). Stories from the WMS subjects were characterized by the abundant use of evaluative devices that served to enrich the referential content of the stories. For instance, subjects with WMS frequently modified their voices to enhance aspects of the story (affective prosody), and made frequent lexically

Increased Evaluation in Adolescents with Williams Syndrome

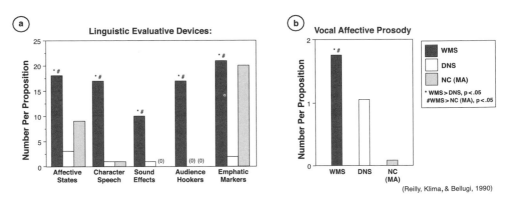

(Reilly, Klima, & Bellugi, 1990)

Figure 2.2
(a) Quantitative analyses reveal that individuals with WMS use significantly more linguistic evaluative devices to enhance their narratives than same-age subjects with DNS or mental age-matched normal controls during the Frog Story task. (b) Vocal affective prosody. Analyses also reveal that vocal affective prosody, such as the use of vocal pitch changes, vocal lengthening, and changes in vocal volume, is used significantly more by WMS than their contrast groups. WMS = Williams Syndrome subjects; DNS = Down Syndrome subjects; NC (MA) = mental age matched normal controls.

encoded inferences about the mental states of the characters they were describing (cognitive evaluation). The WMS stories also included numerous utterances whose sole purpose was to engage the listener. In fact, a new category of measurement called "audience hookers" (a type of social evaluation) was developed for this study because there were frequent instances in which such social evaluative devices were used in WMS stories. For instance, WMS narratives frequently included statements like: ". . . Guess what happened next?," "What do you know?," and "Lo and behold, the frog was gone!" In contrast, DNS narratives were very short and were grammatically impoverished. Moreover, stories from both the DNS and the normally developing children showed little or no evidence of the very high degree of expressiveness both in prosody and in lexical "evaluative" devices evident in the WMS narratives. Figure 2.2 shows the increased affective expression in WMS quantitatively; including linguistically encoded affect and evaluation (a) and exaggerated vocal affective prosody (b). The findings are shown qualitatively as well in Figure 2.3. The contrast in expressivity between the WMS, the DNS, and the normally developing groups provided the first systematic examination of the hypersocial domain in people with WMS.

Social Expression in Story Narratives during Childhood (5–10 years)   The results from the Reilly et al. (1990) study were intriguing, but were limited by small sample sizes, and examined only adolescents with WMS. We initiated a second study with a large sample

Qualitative Examples of Increased Linguistic Evaluation in Adolescents with Williams Syndrome

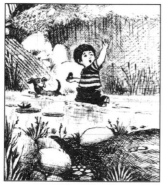

(M. Mayer, "Frog Where are You")

WMS age 13

And he was looking for the frog. What do you know? The frog family! Two lovers. And they were looking. And then he was happy 'cause they had a big family. And said "good bye" and so did the frog. "Ribbit."

WMS age 17

Suddenly when they found the frogs... There was a whole family of frogs... And ah he was amazed! He looked... and he said "Wow, look at these... a female and a male frog and also lots of baby frogs." Then he take one of the little frogs home. So when the frog grow up, it will be his frog... The boy said "Good bye, Mrs. Frog... good bye many frogs. I might see you again if I come around again". "Thank you Mr. Frog and Mrs. Frog for letting me have one of your baby frogs to remember him".

DNS age 13

There you are. Little frog. There another little frog. They in that... water thing. That's it. Frog right there.

DNS age 18

Thy're hiding; see the frogs... the baby frogs. Uh, the boy, and, and the dog saw the frogs. The frog's got babies. The boy saw the... no, the boy say good bye.

(Reilly, Klima & Bellugi, 1990)

Figure 2.3
Qualitative examples from narratives of the "Frog, Where Are You?" story show the excessive use of narrative evaluative devices in adolescents with WMS.

of school-aged children 5–10 years old as a follow up to the original narrative study of adolescents (Bellugi, Losh, Reilly, & Anderson, 1998; Losh, Reilly, Bellugi, Cassady, & Klima, 1997; Jones, Bellugi, Harrison, Rossen, & Klima, 1995). The results from this study of developing WMS children are presented here. Using a narrative task, the performance of young school-aged children with WMS was compared to that of age- and gender-matched normal controls.

SUBJECTS.   The Frog Story task was administered to 30 children with WMS (mean age 7.8 years; range 5–10 years) and 30 age- and gender-matched normal control children (mean age 7.8 years; range 5–10 years).

PROCEDURES.   The study involved the wordless picture book called "Frog, Where Are You?" (Mayer, 1969), a book that describes a boy and his dog looking for their lost frog. Subjects were asked to produce a narrative on the basis of pictures from the book. Narratives were video-recorded and transcribed by trained coders using the MinCHAT program (MacWhinney, 1995). Each transcript was coded for the number of clauses, morphosyntactic errors, sentence complexity, uses of vocal prosody, and the use of evaluative devices. Indices of vocal prosody included the use of vocal lengthening (saying, "Oh, Mr. Fro*ooooooooo*g"). Evaluative devices included exclamatory phrases that functioned to renew and maintain audience attention, character speech, or sound effects. These were frequently accompanied by exclamatory vocal prosody (and seemed to serve to hold the audience's attention), devices that we have termed social engagement devices or audience hookers. Examples from stories of WMS abound: "*Lo and behold!* He knew why his frog had run away. It was time for him to have children . . . ," "Suddenly he woke up." Also noted were the following evaluative devices: 1) The subject inferred the emotional state of a story character ("He was *sad* because the frog left"); 2) Emphatic markers to dramatize the story ("He was *really* sad"); and 3) Inferences of character motivation, causality or mental states ("He *thinks* the frog might be under the log"). We termed the latter *cognitive interferences*.

Because subjects told stories of varying lengths, each index was calculated as a ratio of the total number of propositions used. For instance, the number of times a child used vowel lengthening in their story was divided by the number of proposition (defined as a phrase including a verb and its complements). Data were analyzed with analysis of variance, using group as a factor and with specific measures (e.g., number of propositions, number of exclamatory phrases, etc.) used as dependent variables.

RESULTS.   The children with WMS made significantly more morphological errors than their normal controls (ANOVA with proportion of errors by group: $F(2,57) = 21.9, p < .05$). These error findings were not surprising, considering the language and cognitive delays seen in early development in WMS. However, like their adolescent counterparts,

High Levels of Evaluation in Young Children with Williams Syndrome (5–10 years)

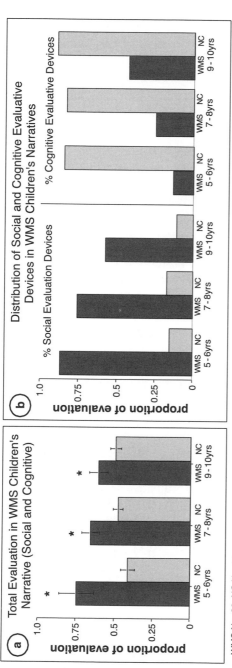

WMS N = 30, NC N = 30
* WMS> NC (CA), p<.05

Figure 2.4

(a) Total evaluation in WMS children's narrative (social and cognitive). Young children with WMS make many more morphosyntactic errors in narratives and, yet, consistently use abnormally high levels of linguistic evaluation in their Frog Story narratives when compared to same-age normal controls. (b) Abnormally, high use of Social Evaluative Devices in WMS children's narratives. WMS children (5–10) make excessive use of socially engaging comments at the expense of using cognitive devices at every age level. They show strong predilection for using social evaluation in their stories, reflecting their hypersociability in language from an early age. NC = normal controls; WMS = Williams Syndrome subjects.

young children with WMS made extensive use of evaluative devices to elaborate their stories (ANOVA with total linguistic evaluative devices by group: $F(2,57) = 22.9$, $p <$ .05); (see Figure 2.4a). When we look internally at the distribution of the different types of evaluation employed (e.g., social vs. cognitive evaluations, as in Figure 2.4b), the young WMS children also greatly exceeded normal controls in their use of social engagement devices (ANOVA with social engagement devices by group: $F(2,57) = 27.8$, $p < .05$). Conversely, controls used a higher proportion of inferences of characters' cognitive states or motivations (ANOVA with all cognitive evaluation devices by group: $F(2,57) = 24.8$, $p < .05$). When these effects were examined by age, the children with WMS used more social evaluative devices across all age groups (all comparisons significant at $p < .05$), and used fewer cognitive evaluative devices than the normal controls (all comparisons significant at $p < .05$).

DISCUSSION.   As we might predict from the studies on early language development in WMS children, this group of young children made more errors than their normally developing peers. In great contrast, the WMS stories were consistently high in the total instances of evaluative devices (including intensifiers, character motivation and affective states, and the use of phrases and exclamations to capture audience attention). Despite their late language acquisition and frequent grammatical errors in their stories, even the youngest children with WMS used linguistically encoded evaluation more than normal controls. In addition to these group differences showing the high frequency of use of evaluation in WMS, we note that in absolute terms, every individual WMS child in our group exhibited a profile of higher use of evaluative devices than their normal counterparts. This consistency in the high use of evaluation (i.e., lack of variability) stands in stark contrast to the use of evaluation in normally developing children as well as to WMS subjects' performance on structural measures of language. While normally developing children use evaluation for more cognitively based inferences, the WMS children, beginning at an early age, used evaluative devices to engage and maintain their listeners' attention. Taken together, these results demonstrate that from the outset WMS children exploit their developing language abilities for social purposes.

Social Expression in a Biographical Interview Task   WMS children and adolescents exploit the potential of narratives by using high levels of affective prosody and lexically encoded evaluative devices in structured storytelling situations as shown above. The question arises as to the generalizability of these findings to other discourse situations. To complement the narrative data, the spontaneous social use of language was examined during a Biographical Interview task administered as a warm-up task during the first meeting with an experimental subject (Harrison, Reilly, & Klima, 1995; Reilly, Harrison, & Klima, 1995). Data from age-matched adolescents and adults with WMS and

DNS were compared to data from normal control individuals matched for approximate developmental age. Subjects were questioned about their interests and activities (pets, siblings, favorite events) in conversational format.

SUBJECTS.   Ten adolescents and adults with WMS and ten with DNS were included in the Biographical Interview study, and were compared to eight normal control subjects matched for approximate developmental age as assessed in previous studies (mean age WMS = 15.8 years, mean age DNS = 15.1 years, mean age controls = 6.5 years).

PROCEDURES.   An experimenter conducted a semistructured interview that involved asking each subject questions about his or her family, activities, and interests. Follow-up questions were asked as consistent with natural conversational flow. The interviews were videotaped and transcribed, and the transcripts were coded for the same evaluative devices examined in the narrative studies above. As with the story narrative study, interview indices were normalized for number of propositions. ANOVA techniques were utilized for examining the data.

RESULTS.   ANOVA with group as a factor showed that adolescents with WMS, DNS and their developmental age-matched controls answered the same number of interview questions ($F(2,25) = .47$, n.s.), and generated equivalent numbers of propositions in response to the questions ($F(2,25) = 1.55$, n.s.). However, there were significant group differences in the total number of lexical evaluative devices used in responses (all devices summed together by experimental group: $F(2,25) = 8.54$, $p = .002$). Post hoc follow-up comparisons revealed that subjects with WMS used significantly more evaluative de-

Converging Evidence from Biographical Interviews

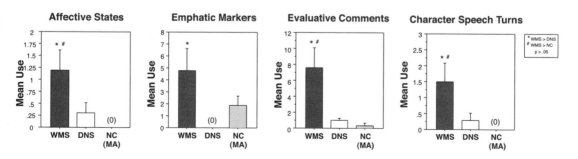

Figure 2.5
Adolescents and adults with WMS use abnormally high levels of social evaluative devices during an interview task, sometimes turning the tables on the examiner and asking him/her questions, while the same-age subjects with DNS or mental age-matched normal controls use little or no affective expression during the task. WMS = Williams Syndrome subjects; DNS = Down Syndrome subjects; NC (MA) = mental age matched normal controls.

vices in their responses than either DNS ($p < .001$) or developmental age-matched normal controls ($p < .01$). In particular, the WMS subjects used more descriptions of affective states, evaluative comments, emphatic markers, and character speech than the DNS or normal control subjects (all differences significant at $p < .05$); (see Figure 2.5).

Additionally, qualitative differences between the WMS interviews and the interviews from other groups were found. For instance, when asked about incidents and facts from their lives, many WMS individuals "turned the tables" on the examiner and actively sought information from them, as if interviewing the examiner. When asked what types of pets he had at home, one WMS subject said, "I have a dog. Do you have a dog? What kind of dog?" Another one asked, "What's your favorite singer?" and another "How long have you lived in California? Where were you born?" Although the interviewer provided brief responses and attempted to redirect the subject to talk about himself or herself, the WMS subjects sometimes continued to ask questions of the experimenter, perhaps a manifestation of the desire for continued social interaction. Finally, when asked to tell about their favorite event, several WMS individuals said something like: "Being here is the best thing that ever happened to me."

DISCUSSION.   The results from this study suggest that subjects with WMS use expressive devices across a number of linguistic settings. They support the previous finding that subjects with WMS use more evaluative devices than other subject groups, and show that this aspect of the social profile extends from the more highly structured narrative to the more conversational context of the interview.

In sum, the results from the studies in Section I demonstrate that subjects with WMS use significantly more evaluative devices than other subject groups, including people with DNS or normal controls. Looking at the function of these evaluative devices, children with WMS used a preponderance of social engagement devices, in contrast to normal control children. The extensive use of social evaluative devices and linguistically encoded affect by WMS subjects is also seen in structured interview tasks as well as in narrative tasks. This is the first empirically driven index of the excessive social and linguistic nature that appears to be a characteristic feature of the WMS phenotype. Taken together, these results demonstrate the pervasiveness of linguistically conveyed hypersociability in WMS.

Section II. Early Development of the Social Nature of WMS

The WMS population is often characterized as unusually social in that subjects exhibit increased interest in engaging others and an apparent ease of engagement in many aspects of the social interaction. For instance, a deaf researcher at The Salk Institute once provided her observation of the differences between WMS and DNS individuals when they come into the lab and up to her desk. Her observation (expressed in sign language) points to the strong drive in children with WMS to engage in social interaction, even in the absence of direct two-way conversation.

The DNS children sometimes come up and touch everything on my desk, so I have to call the experimenter to take them away. The WMS children, in contrast, typically come right up close to me, look me in the face, smile broadly at me, and talk to me even though I sign to them that I can't hear or speak. They seem to be fascinated, continuing to smile and talk to me, all the time looking right into my face while they try to imitate my signs.

This anecdote illustrates the strong attraction to social interaction in children with WMS even when they didn't understand the signed message. The studies presented in Section II focus on very young children with WMS and the emergence of hypersociability.

Until recently, little was known about the early development of sociability in WMS, although this is a behavioral domain of special interest given findings with adolescents and adults with the disorder. Developmentally, the onset of first words and other linguistic and nonlinguistic milestones are significantly delayed in children with the disorder, and it is not until WMS children reach school age that language typically becomes a relative strength (Singer-Harris, Bellugi, Bates, Jones, & Rossen, 1997). Similarly, significant delays in visuospatial and motor abilities, as well as general cognitive development, are seen in infants and young children (Jones et al., 1999a; Jones, Lai, & Bellugi, 1999b). The observed delays in these aspects of development raises questions of whether the WMS hypersociability appears late, together with the onset of language, or whether it is present prelingually. The early presence of a special hypersocial personality could suggest that this aspect of the WMS phenotype may be independent of other cognitive abilities and is pervasive across development, representing a persistent trait throughout the age span in people with WMS.

Section II presents a study that was designed to measure frequency and intensity of emotional expression as an index for early social behavior (Jones, Anderson, Reilly, & Bellugi, 1998). Using infants and toddlers with WMS (subjects younger than 5 years of age), the study investigates the extent to which the hypersocial nature is present during early development in WMS, or if development in this behavioral domain is delayed similarly to other aspects of cognition. For the study, infants and toddlers with WMS were matched to normal controls matched for developmental or chronological age. Children were administered a subset of the Laboratory Temperament Assessment Battery (LabTab), a battery that was developed to assess positive and negative emotional expression in young children (Goldsmith & Rothbart, 1991, 1992).

SUBJECTS.   Twenty-two WMS children aged 15 to 58 months were matched on developmental age and gender to 22 normal controls (mean age WMS = 18.5 months; mean age controls = 18.2 months). In addition, 14 WMS children aged 15 to 31 months were matched on chronological age and gender to 14 normal controls (mean age WMS = 24.6 months; mean age controls = 22.2 months). Results from t tests revealed that the groups were well matched for developmental or chronological age (all tests n.s. at $p = .05$).

PROCEDURES.   The Parental Separation task from the LabTab (Goldsmith & Rothbart, 1991, 1992) was used as an index of emotional expression. The LabTab is a structured series of tasks developed to elicit specific emotional responses in young children. The Parental Separation task was designed to elicit anger, frustration, and then happiness, and began with the child and parent playing quietly on the floor with specific toys. After 3 to 5 min of free play, the parent was instructed to say "goodbye" to the child and then to leave the room. The child was left alone in the room and was watched closely from behind a one-way mirror. After 30–60 sec the child was reunited with the parent. Affective responses on the face, through the voice, and on the body were coded according to LabTab criteria (Goldsmith & Rothbart, 1992). Frequency and intensity of each behavior was recorded.

Positive and negative facial expressions were coded during the separation period, and included the presence of either sad, angry, or happy expressions on the face. Vocal behaviors were coded as well, and included crying, whining, whimpering, screaming, cooing, or cheering. Frequencies of each of these affective expressions during the separation period were recorded. Intensity of each expression was tallied on a four-point scale as well, with 0 representing no identifiable expression, and three representing an obvious affective appearance (for instance, an angry facial expression across the eyes, mouth and cheeks). Data were analyzed with repeated measures ANOVA, using group (WMS, normal controls) by condition (face, voice, physical). Positive and negative expressions were examined separately. Comparisons between the WMS subjects and their chronological age-matched controls were conducted separately from comparisons to the developmental age-matched controls, and the frequency and intensity of each condition were analyzed independently as well.

The Bayley Scales of Infant Development (Bayley, 1969) or the Bayley Scales of Infant Development Second Edition (Bayley, 1993) were administered to all children with WMS as an assessment of developmental age (three WMS children were assessed using the original Bayley prior to the release of the second edition). Developmental ages for WMS children above 42 months were calculated using norms for the oldest age group described in the Bayley (1993) manual (42 months). No child with WMS performed at the ceiling or the floor of the Bayley scales, suggesting that the measure adequately measured the cognitive abilities of the children in the study. Cognitive functioning of the control children was assumed to be within normal limits since the children had met criteria for inclusion into the studies as described above.

Emotional Expression in Infants and Children in Parental Separation Task

Frequency of Negative Expressions

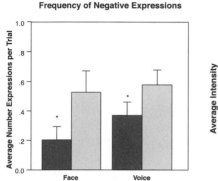

Intensity of Negative Expressions

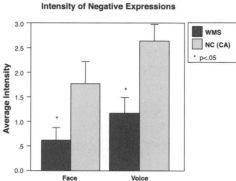

Figure 2.6
Infants and young children with WMS show more positive (e.g., less frequent and less intense negative) emotional expression than chronological age-matched normal controls during a parental separation task. NC (CA) = normal controls (chronological age); WMS = Williams Syndrome subjects.

RESULTS.   During the Parental Separation task in which the child and their parent were purposefully separated, children with WMS expressed less frequent negative facial expressions than chronological age-matched normal controls (repeated measures ANOVA with group by frequency of expression; $F(1,26) = 3.65$, $p < .05$). Moreover, subjects with WMS expressed lower intensity of vocal ($F(1,26) = 5.96$, $p < .05$) and facial ($F(1,26) = 6.06$, $p < .05$) distress and negativity than chronological age-matched controls (see Figure 2.6). These same effects were also found when individuals with WMS were compared to developmental age-matched controls (facial intensity: $F(1,42) = 15.52$, $p < .01$); vocal intensity ($F(1,42) = 11.52$, $p < .01$). Although normal control children in both groups whined, hit objects, or showed clear evidence of frustration during the period of parental separation, the WMS children did so less frequently and less intensely. Instead, the children with WMS played quietly on the floor with their toys, moved toward the door and waited for their parent to return, or explored the room alone with limited negative expression. When reunited with their parents, the WMS children typically re-engaged in play quickly, while the normally developing children frequently needed consoling to continue. In terms of frequency and intensity of positive expression, the children with WMS were the same as control groups on the Parental Separation task ($p < .10$ for all comparisons).

A Young Child Focuses on the Experimenter's Face During Barrier Task

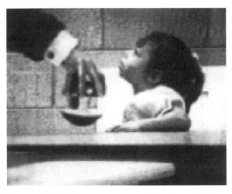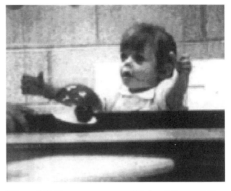

The child ignores toy, looks at the experimenter, beginning of task.

The child's eyes are still looking at the experimenter even when a plexiglass barrier is placed in front of her.

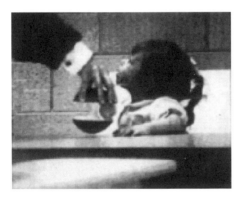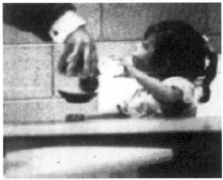

When task is repeated for a second trial, the child again looks up to the experimenter, ignoring the toy.

The child looks at the experimenter, even when the toy is rattled in front of her at the end of the task.

Figure 2.7
A toddler with WMS looks to the experimenter's face at the expense of performing a cognitive task, such as reaching for a toy behind a barrier.

A second important aspect of the early WMS personality appears to include an increased interest in others, as evidenced by the use of positive emotional expressions and/or engaging behaviors directed toward other people. A friendly and overly positive nature was detected during an unstructured warm-up task as well as during standardized cognitive tasks. During the warm-up task, where a child was shown a toy behind a barrier, several WMS children looked excessively at the experimenter's face, often at the expense of performing the task at hand (see Figure 2.7). While the normal children were more likely to kick their feet or hit the barrier, the children with WMS tended to engage the examiner using eye contact and by smiling and sometimes cooing (many were prelingual). The WMS children also tended to use alternate behaviors to occupy their interest (e.g., engaging the experimenter, playing with the edge of the table or waving at their parent), rather than becoming upset as normal young children did if they were unable to complete a task.

In addition, during the IQ test administered to assess developmental age, a large number of WMS subjects demonstrated developmentally abnormal social behaviors. For instance, of the seven children tested on a specific block of Bayley items, five demonstrated such concentrated interest in the examiner's face that it appeared to negatively affect their performance on motoric activities. Instead of watching their hands or the objects as they put blocks in a cup, the WMS children tended to engage the experimenter through eye contact, and then smile at the examiner as they placed the blocks in the cup. This unusual social behavior toward the examiner sometimes resulted in their failing an item of the task because they were interacting with the experimenter, rather than engaging in the task with objects. Few of the WMS subjects became distressed when the tasks were difficult. Instead of pushing blocks away or dropping items on the floor when they were frustrated, the WMS subjects tended to smile at the examiner, look to their parent, or babble at or engage others in the room.

DISCUSSION. The findings from this study are interpreted as support for the early emergence of a hypersocial profile in WMS. The social behavior of infants with the disorder is characterized by a strong attraction to social interaction that may interfere with their focus on cognitively driven tasks. Such behaviors may be used by infants and toddlers with WMS to deflect from engagement in activities that are difficult for them. Behaviors, such as prolonged eye contact and smiling, appear to be used to socially engage others and, yet, may interfere with their ability to respond with appropriate cognitive solutions. The findings suggest that many aspects of the expressive and social nature of people with WMS are present very early on. Together, the results suggest that children with WMS may have an attraction to social interaction, which is apparent even in infancy.

Section III. Hypersociability Toward Strangers as Characteristic of WMS

The social behaviors of individuals with WMS include an apparent lack of fear of strangers and an overfriendliness with strangers. For instance, one mother reported that her daughter with WMS approached a stranger in a department store and asked what she had in her purse. The woman was so taken with the child that she emptied out her entire purse so that the child could view the items! There are consistent reports from parents stating that their WMS child has an almost "uncontrollable urge" to approach people. Similarly, parents often report that their WMS child has an unusual ability to remember the faces and names of individuals that they meet, even for people that they have met only once, years earlier. Often parents cannot recall all the information the child can. Parent anecdotes consistently describe a WMS personality type that is characterized by fearlessness in social interactions with strangers, an excessive desire for social contact, and an ability to readily connect with strangers and engage them in conversation. Section III describes an experiment that quantifies the increased tendency of WMS individuals to approach and engage in interactions with strangers.

SUBJECTS.   Twenty-six subjects with WMS and 26 age- and gender-matched normal controls were included (mean age WMS = 23.6 years, SD = 8.6, 16 female, 10 male; mean age controls = 25.5 years, SD = 7.7, 15 female, 11 male). Results from a t test with age and group revealed that the groups were well matched (n.s., $p > .05$). A third group of 12 normally developing children of ages 7–10 years (mean age 8.3 years) was also included in order to provide a group matched approximately to the general cognitive performance of the WMS group; this group is referred to as "mental-age controls."

STIMULI AND PROCEDURES.   The task included in the study came from a modified version of a task that has been used previously to assess social judgment in adult populations (Adolphs, Tranel, & Damasio, 1998), the Approachability task. For the purposes of the WMS study, this task was slightly altered and the rating scale modified to better accommodate the behavioral and cognitive needs of the WMS subjects. Subjects were shown black-and-white photographs of unfamiliar adult faces in natural poses. Forty-two stimuli from the original 100 photographs used by Adolphs et al. (1998) were selected (the 21 pictures previously found to be rated most approachable, and the 21 previously found to be rated least approachable by normal adult subjects; cf. Adolphs et al., 1998). Upon seeing each photograph, subjects were asked to rate how much they would like to go up to each person and begin a conversation with them. There was no time limit. Response ratings were given on a five-point color-coded Likert scale, with higher scores denoting a greater desire to approach and talk to the person (see Figure 2.8). Each response was coded numerically on a scale from –2 to +2. Before beginning the task, subjects were familiarized with the rating scale using a sample set of faces.

Ratings of Unfamiliar Faces: Approachability Task

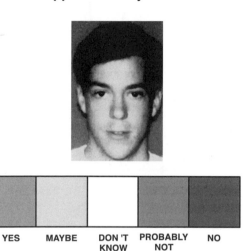

YES	MAYBE	DON 'T KNOW	PROBABLY NOT	NO

Figure 2.8
For the Adolphs' Approachability Rating task, each subject is asked to rate the extent to which they would like to go up and talk to (approach) an unfamiliar person pictured. They rate their responses on a five-point color-coded scale from "definitely yes" to "definitely no."

RESULTS.   We divided our analysis into two parts: Data for the 21 faces that normal controls gave the most negative ratings, and data for the 21 faces that normal controls gave the most positive ratings. An examination of the mean ratings given to each block of 21 faces showed that subjects with WMS gave more positive ratings than did normal subjects. For the 21 most negative faces, WMS subjects gave mean ratings of 0.54 (SD = 1.39) while normal controls gave mean ratings of –0.96 (SD = 0.96); and for the 21 most positive faces, WMS gave mean ratings of 1.32 (SD = 1.1) while normal controls gave mean ratings of 0.84 (SD = 1.12).

ANOVA with subject group (WMS, normal control, mental age control) and stimulus valence (in the 21 most positive faces, or in the 21 most negative faces) as factors was performed. There were significant effects of subject group ($F = 10.67$, $p < .0001$), of stimulus valence ($F = 227.18$, $p < .0001$), and of their interaction ($F = 19.04$, $p < .0001$). Scheffe post hoc tests revealed that the two control groups did not differ ($p > .2$), but that WMS subjects differed significantly from both same age normal controls ($p < .01$) and from mental age controls ($p < .0005$) in giving abnormally positive ratings overall. Post hoc tests of the interaction between subject group and stimulus valence showed

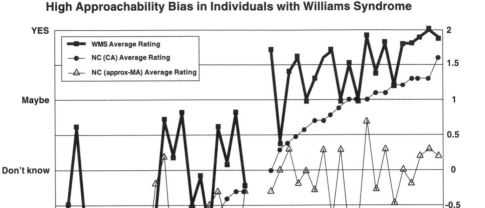

Figure 2.9
In the experimental task, adolescents with WMS consistently rate themselves as more likely to approach and engage unfamiliar individuals than do chronological age-matched normal controls or mental age-matched controls (younger children). NC (CA) = normal controls (chronological age-matched); NC (approx-MA) = normal controls (approximately mental age-matched); WMS = Williams Syndrome subjects.

that subjects with WMS rated the 21 most negative faces significantly more positively than either same age normal controls (mean rating difference = .44; $p < .001$) or mental age controls (mean rating difference = .43, $p < .001$) (see Figure 2.9). The subjects with WMS also rated the 21 most positive faces more positively than either normal controls (mean rating difference = .46; $p < .001$) or mental age controls (mean rating difference = 1.1; $p < .001$). Interestingly, the two control groups did not differ in their ratings of positive faces (mental age controls rated those faces more negatively than normal controls; mean difference = 0.6, $p < .001$). Thus, subjects with WMS gave abnormally positive ratings of approachability to unfamiliar people, compared both to normal controls of the same age, and to normal controls of approximately the same mental age. Taken together, the findings demonstrate an abnormally positive social bias in WMS.

Comments stated by subjects during the task highlight the sociability differences between the groups. For example, one WMS subject commented that a specific face "looked happy, because he's smiling," whereas a normal individual described the same face as having "a mischievous-looking smirk." These types of differences were seen across multiple items of the task, and across subjects in the study. They suggest that individuals with WMS may rely more heavily on superficial signals that are typically viewed positively (e.g., smiling faces), but ignore more subtle social cues (e.g., furrowed eyebrows)—important issues to be addressed in future studies.

DISCUSSION.   The present findings expand and replicate the data from a prior study (Bellugi, Adolphs, Cassady, & Chiles, 1999a), and demonstrate that adolescents and adults with WMS consistently judge unfamiliar individuals as abnormally approachable, consistent with their interest in approaching strangers and engaging them in real life. To our knowledge, these studies are the first to provide a quantitative assessment of the unusual tendency to approach and engage in interactions with strangers in adolescents and adults with WMS. The findings support observations that overfriendliness, as targeted in this study, is characteristic of WMS individuals during real world social interactions. This study provides strong support for hypersociability as a phenotypic feature in individuals with WMS.

Section IV. Contrasting Social Phenotypes: WMS, DNS, and Autism

The sociability exhibited by many WMS individuals is often described by parents as pervasive and seemingly difficult to inhibit, particularly with respect to social approach behaviors to strangers. In great contrast, individuals with autism are typically asocial and tend not to interact with others, whether strangers or not. Thus, individuals with WMS and those with autism represent two polar opposite groups in terms of social behavior. Individuals with DNS have been characterized as friendly, but the similarities and differences between these three groups have not been investigated to date. We designed a study to investigate social behavior in these three contrasting groups.

For this study, an experimental sociability questionnaire was developed to better characterize the limits of the social nature seen in individuals with WMS (Chiles, Bellugi, & Cassady, 1998). On the questionnaire, parents were asked to rate their child's specific social abilities and tendencies. Items assessed the tendency to approach others, general behavior in social situations, ability to remember names and faces, eagerness to please other people, tendency to empathize with or comment on others' emotional states, and the tendency for other people to approach the child. The questionnaire was administered to same-aged subjects with WMS, DNS, and normal controls. In addition, the questionnaire was also administered to same-aged subjects with stringently diagnosed autism (see Figure 2.10), as part of a study in progress. Subjects with autism provide a striking contrast to WMS in terms of social behavior.

SUBJECTS.   The Salk Institute Sociability Questionnaire was sent to 20 parents of individuals with WMS (mean age = 18.9 years; SD = 10.7), 20 parents of individuals with autism (mean age = 17.9 years; SD = 7.1), 20 parents of individuals with DNS (mean age = 18.9 years; SD = 13.0), as well as 15 parents of typically developing children (mean age = 17.0 years; SD = 10.7). Results from ANOVA with age by syndrome revealed that the groups in the study were well matched on age (n.s., $p > .05$).

PROCEDURES.   The Salk Institute Sociability Questionnaire was developed as an index of the many aspects of sociability seen in people with WMS (Chiles et al., 1998). The questionnaire is a parental-report rating scale in which parents are asked to rate their

The Sociability Questionnaire for Williams Syndrome, Down Syndrome, and Autism

"Give some examples of your teenager socializing with strangers:"

WMS	Autistic	DNS
He will go right up to a stranger, get eye contact, and say "hi" again and again until that person says "hi" back.	All people are treated the same-- avoid whenever possible. She will isolate herself and engage in repetitive rituals. She recognizes people but prefers to be alone.	Shy, averts eyes, avoids person, physically withdrawn unless person can communicate with him, then he is engaged easily.
"Hi, my name is B, what is your name?" or "It's nice to meet you, do you own a car wash?" He would always approach the person, introduce himself, and then ask questions.	No speech, head down, very shy and unapproachable.	Mother usually has to initiate and encourage, and then sometimes he will socialize.
Very happy to meet them. Asks many questions about them, their family, pets, language, nationality and number of children.	Requires prompt to say hello. Avoids people whenever possible.	Somewhat quiet and shy, unless he feels comfortable.
"Oh it's so nice to meet you. Where are you from? Are you married? I have a dog, do you have a dog? Oh really?!!! I have a friend who has a broken arm, bad back, new baby, a cat...etc."	Does not socialize with strangers.	Can be shy but appropriate, says "hello."

Figure 2.10
Parents of adolescents and adults with WMS report unusual interest and predilection for approaching others. Typical qualitative examples are shown from each group. The social behavior reported for WMS was in stark contrast to that reported for Autism, and characteristically different (hypersocial) from that reported for DNS and for typically developing normal individuals in the same-age range. DNS = Down Syndrome subjects; WMS = Williams Syndrome subjects.

child's specific social abilities and tendencies on a seven-point Likert scale with low-, mid-, and high-endpoint labels tailored to each individual item. Questionnaire items were designed to measure two aspects of sociability: Social approach behavior and social emotional behavior. The items that measure social approach behavior consist of statements such as "Compare your child's tendency to approach strangers with an average child of the same age," and "Compare a stranger's tendency to engage your child with an average child of the same age." Other questionnaire items were designed to assess their social-emotional behavior. These items measure their tendency to empathize with or comment on other people's emotional state, as well as the accuracy of their emotional evaluation of others and their eagerness to please other people. In addition, parents are also asked to provide qualitative descriptions of their child in various social situations.

Three composite scores were developed on the basis of the original questionnaire items: (A) The Global Sociability score combines the scores of all items on the questionnaire and is designed as a cross-domain measure of Sociability; (B) the Social Approach score combines only the scores of items related to the subject's approach behavior toward other people (e.g., tendency to approach strangers); and (C) the Social Emotional score is composed of the items querying social behaviors, such as the accuracy of their emotional evaluation of others. ANOVA were used for all comparisons, with group as a factor, and each composite score as a dependent measure.

RESULTS.   Qualitative examples from the questionnaire items highlight the differences between the WMS, Autism, and DNS groups. For example, when asked to give an ex-

Quantitative Measures of Sociability Contrasting Williams Syndrome, Down Syndrome, and Autism

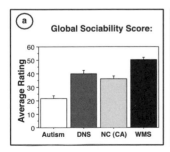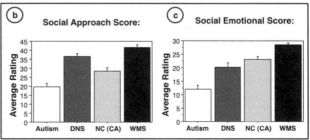

Figure 2.11
Individuals with WMS are consistently rated as more social than individuals with Autism, DNS, or normal controls matched for chronological age on several parental report scales of social behavior, including Global Sociability behaviors as well as Social Approach and Social Emotional items. NC (CA) = normal controls (chronological age); WMS = Williams Syndrome subjects; DNS = Down Syndrome subjects.

ample of their children socializing with strangers, the parent of an Autistic adolescent said, "[He] requires a prompt to say hello. [He] avoids people whenever possible." The parent of a same-age DNS adolescent said, "[He is] somewhat quiet and shy unless he feels comfortable." In contrast, the parent of an adolescent with WMS reported, "[He] is very happy to meet people. [He] asks many questions about them, their family, pets, language, nationality and number of children." See Figure 2.10 for additional examples.

ANOVA with group (WMS, DNS, autism and normal control) by Global Sociability score revealed significant differences between the groups on this measure ($F(3,59) =$ 31.11, $p < .0001$). Post hoc follow-up comparisons revealed that subjects with WMS were rated as being significantly more social than were the DNS, autistic or normal control subjects (all comparisons $p < .001$), while autistic subjects were rated least social relative to the other groups ($p < .001$). DNS subjects and normal controls were rated comparably by their parents ($p > .20$) and had mean scores between the WMS and autistic groups (see Figure 2.11a). Examples of parental comments characterize the typical differences among the groups.

Breaking down the general sociability findings, specific subcategories of differences were also found. A significant difference between the groups was detected for the Social-Emotional subscale ($F(3,60) = 31.08, p < .0001$). Follow-up comparisons revealed that the WMS group was consistently rated higher than the autistic group on this scale as well and, indeed, scored the highest of all the reference groups on the Social-Emotional subscale (all comparisons significant, $p < .01$; see Figure 2.11b). In addition, the autistic group was consistently rated lower than the other groups (all comparisons significant, $p < .0001$), while the DNS and normal control groups were rated similarly by their parents (n.s., $p > .05$).

Significant differences among the groups were also found for a scale measuring Social Approach behaviors ($F(3,65) = 30.06, p < .0001$). Subjects with WMS were rated most highly in their interest in approaching others (all comparisons significant, $p < .05$), while subjects with autism were rated the lowest (all comparisons significant, $p < .01$). Subjects with DNS were rated more highly than normal controls and subjects with autism, but were rated lower than subjects with WMS (all comparisons significant, $p < .05$); while normal controls were rated significantly higher than subjects with autism, but were lower than the WMS and DNS groups (all comparisons significant, $p < .05$).

DISCUSSION.   The findings from this study support previous results related to a social profile in WMS. The profile appears to consist of an excessive interest in others and a lack of inhibition toward approaching other individuals. As expected, subjects with autism are judged to have significant social deficits and appear uninterested in approaching others. Normal control and DNS subjects are social but not overly so, while WMS subjects are generally overly social and exhibit a tendency to hypersociability. The findings suggest that WMS behavior within the domain of sociability may be distinct from that seen in other disorders. Such findings provide the framework for investigating the neurobiological basis of social behavior.

The findings from the study also demonstrate specific differences in sociability between individuals with WMS and those with other disorders, notably those with autism. Indeed, social behavioral contrasts between WMS and autism are striking (Courchesne, Bellugi, & Singer, 1995). WMS children seek out social interaction and eye contact and, generally, do it in a polite and friendly manner. Galaburda, Wang, Bellugi, and Rossen (1994) write in a description of a WMS child, "He drew people to him as though he had a (social) magnet in him." In contrast, the cardinal feature of autism is a profound deficiency in social knowledge, affective expression, and communication. The autistic child avoids eye contact and is poor at discriminating facial expressions. In an early description of an autistic child, Kanner (1943) wrote, "He paid no attention to persons around him . . . he completely disregarded the people (in a room) and instantly went for an object . . . he was happiest when left alone." Future studies examining the neuroanatomical differences between WMS and Autism may reveal clues to aspects of the neural and genetic bases of social behavior.

Conclusion

The studies reported in this chapter show that hypersociability is a salient aspect of behavior in WMS. The WMS social nature consists of a strong drive toward social interaction with other people. As Section I shows, the social drive appears to influence other cognitive domains, including language, and evidence of it can be detected even in simple narrative and storytelling tasks. Section II suggests that it is developmentally pervasive, as evidence of it is detected in children even before they are able to talk. Sections III and IV suggest that it is quantifiable through both objective tasks, such as those measuring subjective interest in approaching other people, as well as through parental report. Finally, Section IV reveals that the hypersocial drive of subjects with WMS appears to strongly distinguish WMS from other disorders, including autism and DNS, as well as from normally developing peers. Taken together, the studies presented here suggest that the social behavior of subjects with WMS is quantifiable and, indeed, highly unusual relative to other disorders. The findings now prepare future studies linking this aspect of the WMS phenotype to other domains, including genetics and neuroanatomy.

Current studies of brain morphology in WMS are progressing rapidly and are likely to lead to the neurobiological underpinnings of the behaviors described in this study (see, for instance, Galaburda & Bellugi, chap. 5; Reiss et al., chap. 4; Jernigan, Bellugi, Sowell, Doherty, & Hesselink, 1993). The amygdala, for instance, has been found to play a role in social behavior and may be a likely neurological substrate for some of the behaviors described in WMS. Like patients with focal bilateral damage to the amygdala (Adolphs et al., 1998), individuals with WMS give abnormally positive ratings to unfamiliar people, appear unusually friendly, and tend to approach others somewhat indiscriminately in real life. However, there are also notable differences between the performances given by subjects with WMS and those previously reported for subjects with bilateral amygdala damage. Importantly, subjects with WMS gave abnormally positive ratings across all faces. Subjects with amygdala damage, in contrast, were found to give more positive ratings only for faces that typically received the most negative ratings from controls (Adolphs et al., 1998). Taken together, the findings may suggest links between aspects of abnormal social behavior in WMS, and possible dysfunction in the amygdala and other limbic regions.

The WMS social profile also provides an opportunity for scientists to hypothesize about new brain areas underlying aspects of social behavior. It was not until recently, for example, that the role of the cerebellum was expanded from motor behavior to also encompass aspects of higher cognition. Studies now suggest, for example, that the cerebellum may play a role in regulating affective expression across various disorders (Schmahmann, 1997; Schmahmann & Sherman, 1998). Neuroanatomical contrasts between subjects with WMS and Autism suggest that areas of the cerebellum may play a role in the sociability differences between these two disorders. Whereas the neocerebellar vermis appears to be disproportionately enlarged in individuals with WMS (Jones et al., 1999b; Wang, Hesselink, Jernigan, Doherty, & Bellugi, 1992), it appears disproportionately small in individuals with autism and may be one important substrate of the social deficiencies in the disorder (Courchesne et al., 1994a; Courchesne, Townsend, & Saitoh, 1994b). Such contrasts between WMS and other disorders are likely to lead to better delineation of the neurological bases of social behavior.

The work described in this chapter highlights a new aspect of the WMS phenotype. Taken in combination with other behaviors in the syndrome, the phenotype is providing the pathway for linking specific genes to specific behaviors, as well as to the specific brain areas underlying these behaviors. By adding a new dimension to the previously described phenotype in WMS, the studies described here provide a more specific behavioral profile to better guide studies of the anatomic and genetic underpinnings of WMS. We pursue the study of social behavior in WMS with the aim of linking findings to brain morphology and, ultimately, to the gene.

Notes

The research was supported by grants from the National Institute of Child Health and Human Development (P01 HD33113 to Ursula Bellugi, PD), the National Institute of Deafness and Communication Disorders (P50 DC01289, Project 3 to Ursula Bellugi, PI), and the National Institute of Neurological Disorders and Strokes (P50 NS22343, Project 3 to Ursula Bellugi, PI), The Oak Tree Philanthropic Foundation, and the James S. McDonnell Foundation.The authors thank the Regional and National Williams syndrome Associations and the individuals with Williams syndrome who participated in these studies. The authors are grateful to Edward S. Klima for his helpful comments.

Illustrations and quotes not to be used without written permission from the author. Copyright Dr. Ursula Bellugi, La Jolla, CA.

References

Adolphs, R., Tranel, D., & Damasio, A. (1998). The human amygdala in social judgment. *Nature, 393,* 470–474.

Bamburg, M., & Reilly, J. (1996). Emotion, narrative and affect: How children discover the relationship between what to say and how to say it. In D. Slobin, J. Gerhardt, A. Kyratzis, & J. Guo (Eds.), *Interaction, social context, and language: Essays in honor of Susan Ervin-Tripp* (pp. 329–342). Hillsdale, NJ: Erlbaum.

Bayley, N. (1969). *Bayley scales of infant development.* Princeton, NJ: Psychological Corporation.

Bayley, N. (1993). *The Bayley scales of infant development* (2nd ed.). San Antonio, TX: Psychological Corporation.

Bellugi, U., Adolphs, R., Cassady, C., & Chiles, M. (1999a). Towards the neural basis for hypersociability in a genetic syndrome. *NeuroReport, 10,* 1–5.

Bellugi, U., Lichtenberger, L., Jones, W., Lai, Z., & St. George, M. (chap. 1). The neurocognitive profile of Williams Syndrome: A complex pattern of strengths and weaknesses.

Bellugi, U., Lichtenberger, L., Mills, D., Galaburda, A., & Korenberg, J. (1999b). Bridging cognition, brain and molecular genetics: Evidence from Williams syndrome. *Trends in Neurosciences, 22,* 197–207.

Bellugi, U., Losh, M., Reilly, J., & Anderson, D. (1998). Excessive use of linguistically encoded affect: Stories from young children with Williams syndrome. Technical report CND-9801. University of California at San Diego, Center for Research in Language, Project of Cognitive and Neural Development.

Bellugi, U., Mills, D., Jernigan, T., Hickok, G., & Galaburda, A. (1999c). Linking cognition, brain structure and brain function in Williams syndrome. In H. Tager-Flusberg (Ed.), *Neurodevelopmental disorders: Contributions to a new framework from the cognitive neurosciences* (pp. 111–136). Cambridge, MA: MIT Press.

Chiles, M., Bellugi, U., & Cassady, C. (1998). *The sociability questionnaire.* Unpublished test protocol. La Jolla, CA: Laboratory for Cognitive Neuroscience, The Salk Institute for Biological Studies.

Courchesne, E., Saitoh, O., Yeung-Courchesne, R., Press, G., Lincoln, A., Haas, R., & Schreibman, L. (1994a). Abnormality of cerebellar vermian lobules VI and VII in patients with infantile autism: Identification of hypoplastic and hyperplastic subgroups with MR imaging. *American Journal of Roentgenology, 163,* 123–130.

Courchesne, E., Bellugi, U., & Singer, N. (1995). Infantile autism and Williams syndrome: Social and neural worlds apart. In J. P. Fryns (Ed.), Abstracts from the Williams Syndrome Association Professional Conference [Special Issue]. *Genetic Counseling, 6,* 144–145.

Courchesne, E., Townsend, J., & Saitoh, O. (1994b). The brain in infantile autism: Posterior fossa structures are abnormal. *Neurology, 44,* 214–223.

Einfeld, S., Tonge, B., & Florio, T. (1997). Behavioral and emotional disturbance in individuals with Williams syndrome. *American Journal of Mental Retardation, 102,* 45–53.

Ewart, A., Morris, C., Atkinson, D., Jin, W., Sternes, K., Spallone, P., Stock, A., Leppert, M., & Keating, M. (1993). Hemizygosity at the elastin locus in a developmental disorder, Williams-Beuren syndrome. *Nature Genetics, 5,* 11–16.

Galaburda, A., & Bellugi, U. (chap. 5). Multi-level analysis of cortical neuroanatomy in Williams syndrome.

Galaburda, A., Wang, P., Bellugi, U., & Rossen, M. (1994). Cytoarchitectonic findings in a genetically based disorder: Williams syndrome. *NeuroReport, 5,* 758–787.

Goldsmith, H., & Rothbart, M. (1991). Contemporary instruments for assessing early temperament by questionnaire and in the laboratory. In J. Strelau, & A. Angleitner (Eds.), *Explorations in temperament* (pp. 249–286). New York: Plenum.

Goldsmith, H., & Rothbart, M. (1992). *The laboratory temperament assessment battery: Locomotor version.* Unpublished test manual. Eugene, OR: Department of Psychology, University of Oregon.

Harrison, D., Reilly, J., & Klima, E. (1995). Unusual social behavior in Williams syndrome: Evidence from biographical interviews. *Genetic Counseling, 6,* 181–183.

Jernigan, T., Bellugi, U., Sowell, E., Doherty, S., & Hesselink, J. (1993). Cerebral morphological distinctions between Williams and Down syndromes. *Archives of Neurology, 50,* 186–191.

Jones, W., Anderson, D., Reilly, J., & Bellugi, U. (1998). Emotional expression in infants and children with Williams syndrome: A relationship between temperament and genetics? *Journal of the International Neuropsychological Society, 4,* 56.

Jones, W., Bellugi, U., Harrison, D., Rossen, M. L., & Klima, E. S. (1995, March). Discourse in two genetically based syndromes with contrasting brain anomalies. Paper presented at the meeting of the Society for Research in Child Development, Indianapolis, IN.

Jones, W., Hickok, G., Rossen, M., & Bellugi, U. (1999a, submitted). Dissociations in cognitive development: Evidence from Williams syndrome. *Developmental Neuropsychology.*

Jones, W., Lai, Z. L., & Bellugi, U. (1999b). Relations between cerebellar vermal areas and neuropsychological performance in Williams syndrome. *Journal of the International Neuropsychological Society, 5,* 152.

Kanner, L. (1943). Autistic disturbances of affective contact. *Nervous Child, 2,* 217–250.

Korenberg, J., Chen, X. -N., Hirota, H., Lai, Z., Bellugi, U., Burian, D., Roe, B., & Matsuoka, R. (chap. 6). Genome structure and cognitive map of Williams Syndrome.

Korenberg, J., Chen, X. -N., Mitchell, S., Sun, Z., Hubert, R., Vataru, E., & Bellugi, U. (1996). The genomic organization of Williams syndrome. *American Journal of Medical Genetics, Supplement, 59,* A306, 1776.

Labov, W., & Waletsky, J. (1967). Narrative analysis: Oral versions of personal experience. In J. Helm (Ed.), *Essays on the verbal and visual arts* (pp. 17–35). Seattle, WA: University of Washington Press.

Losh, M., Reilly, J., Bellugi, U., Cassady, C., & Klima, E. (1997). Linguistically encoded affect is abnormally high in Williams syndrome children. *International Behavioral Neuroscience Society Abstracts, 6,* 2–53.

MacWhinney, B. (1995). *The CHILDES project: Tools for analyzing talk* (2nd ed.). Hillsdale, NJ: Erlbaum.

Mayer, M. (1969). *Frog, where are you?* New York, NY: Dial Books for Young Readers.

Mervis, C., Morris, C., Bertrand, J., & Robinson, B. (1999). Williams syndrome: Findings from an integrated program of research. In H. Tager-Flusberg (Ed.), *Neurodevelopmental disorders: Contributions to a new framework from the cognitive neurosciences* (pp. 65–110). Cambridge, MA: MIT Press.

Morris, C., Demsey, S., Leonard, C., Dilts, C., & Blackburn, B. (1988). Natural history of Williams syndrome: Physical characteristics. *Journal of Pediatrics, 113,* 318–326.

Preus, M. (1984). The Williams syndrome: Objective definition and diagnosis. *Journal of Clinical Genetics, 25,* 422–428.

Reilly, J., Harrison, D., & Klima, E. (1995). Emotional talk and talk about emotions. Abstract, *Genetic Counseling, 6,* 181–183.

Reilly, J., Klima, E. S., & Bellugi, U. (1990). Once more with feeling: Affect and language in atypical populations. *Development and Psychopathology, 2,* 367–391.

Reiss, A., Eliez, S., Schmitt, J. E., Strous, E., Lai, Z., Jones, W., & Bellugi, U. (chap. 4). Neuroanatomy of Williams syndrome: A high-resolution MRI study.

Rossen, M., Klima, E. S., Bellugi, U., Bihrle, A., & Jones, W. (1996). Interaction between language and cognition: Evidence from Williams syndrome. In J. H. Beitchman, N. Cohen, M. Konstantareas, & R. Tannock (Eds.), *Language, learning, and behavior disorders: Developmental, biological, and clinical perspectives* (pp. 367–392). New York, NY: Cambridge University Press.

Schmahmann, S. D. (1997). *The cerebellum and cognition.* San Diego, CA: Academic Press.

Schmahmann, S. D., & Sherman, J. C. (1998). The cerebellar cognitive affective syndrome. *Brain, 121,* 561–579.

Schopler, E., Reichler, R., DeVellis, R., & Daly, K. (1980). Toward objective classification of childhood autism: Childhood Autism Rating Scale (CARS). *Journal of Autism and Developmental Disorders, 10,* 91–103.

Singer-Harris, N. G., Bellugi, U., Bates, E., Jones, W., & Rossen, M. L. (1997). Contrasting profiles of language development in children with Williams and Down syndromes. In D. J. Thal & J. S. Reilly (Eds.), Origins of language disorders [Special Issue]. *Developmental Neuropsychology, 13,* 345–370.

Tager-Flusberg, H., Sullivan, K., Boshart, J., Guttman, J., & Levine, K. (1996, July). Social cognitive abilities in children and adolescents with Williams syndrome. Paper presented at the Seventh International Professional Conference on Williams Syndrome, King of Prussia, PA.

VanLieshout, C., DeMeyer, R., Curfs, L., & Fryns, J. (1998). Family contexts, parental behavior, and personality profiles of children and adolescents with Prader-Willi, Fragile-X, or Williams syndrome. *Journal of Child Psychology and Psychiatry and Allied Disciplines, 39,* 699–710.

Wang, P. P., Hesselink, J. R., Jernigan, T. L., Doherty, S., & Bellugi, U. (1992). The specific neurobehavioral profile of Williams syndrome is associated with neocerebellar hemispheric preservation. *Neurology, 42,* 1999–2002.

3 Neurophysiological Markers of Face Processing in Williams Syndrome

Debra L. Mills, Twyla D. Alvarez, Marie St. George, Lawrence G. Appelbaum, Ursula Bellugi, and Helen Neville

Williams Syndrome (WMS) is a genetically based disorder characterized by pronounced variability in performance across different domains of cognitive functioning. This study examined brain activity linked to face-processing abilities, which are typically spared in individuals with WMS. Subjects watched photographic pairs of upright or inverted faces and indicated if the second face matched or did not match the first face. Results from a previous study with normal adults showed dramatic differences in the timing and distribution of ERP effects linked to recognition of upright and inverted faces. In normal adults, upright faces elicited ERP differences to matched vs. mismatched faces at approximately 320 msec (N320) after the onset of the second stimulus. This "N320" effect was largest over anterior regions of the right hemisphere. In contrast, the mismatch/match effect for inverted faces consisted of a large positive component between 400 and 1000 msec (P500) that was largest over parietal regions and was symmetrical. In contrast to normal adults, WMS subjects showed an N320-mismatch effect for both upright and inverted faces. Additionally, the WMS subjects did not display the N320 right-hemisphere asymmetry observed in the normal adults. WMS subjects also displayed an abnormally small negativity at 100 msec (N100) and an abnormally large negativity at 200 msec (N200) to both upright and inverted faces. This ERP pattern was observed in all subjects with WMS but was not observed in the normal controls. These results may be linked to increased attention to faces in subjects with WMS and might be specific to the disorder. These results were consistent with our ERP studies of language processing in WMS, which suggested abnormal cerebral specialization for spared cognitive functions in individuals with WMS.

Introduction

The relative influence of genetic, maturational, and experiential factors on the development of cerebral specialization is a central issue in cognitive neuroscience. The unusual neurocognitive and genetic profiles in Williams Syndrome (WMS) provide an opportunity to examine how these factors interact to shape cerebral specializations for language and non-language cognitive functions. Williams syndrome is a genetically based disorder characterized by remarkable sparing in some domains, such as language and face recognition, in contrast with marked deficits in other domains, such as spatial abilities (see Bellugi, Lichtenberger, Jones, Lai, & St. George, chap. 1). This disorder is also associated with concomitant abnormalities in brain structure, such as curtailment of the posterior-parietal and occipital regions (see Galaburda & Bellugi, chap. 5; Reiss et al., chap. 4). One approach to studying structure-function relations would be to link abnormalities in brain structure with specific cognitive deficits. For example, deficits in spatial abilities may be linked with abnormal structure (Galaburda & Bellugi, chap. 5) and abnormal function (Atkinson, Braddick, Nokes, Anker, & Braddick, 1997) in the dorsal-visual stream. However, this approach does not provide information about the organization of spared cognitive functions such as language and face processing.

In early neuroanatomical studies, MRI analyses of individuals with WMS suggested normal volumetric measures of frontal and cerebellar structures, which might underlie spared language abilities (Jernigan & Bellugi, 1994). The volume of gray matter in the inferior-posterior medial cortex was positively correlated with face-recognition abilities in individuals with WMS (Jones, Rossen, Hickok, Jernigan, & Bellugi, 1995). Of particular interest was whether a configuration of relatively normal brain structure in regions typically associated with the spared cognitive abilities would be indicative of normal brain function in WMS, as suggested by Bellugi, Mills, Jernigan, Hickok, and Galaburda (1999b). Alternatively, the brain systems that underlie the spared cognitive functions might be abnormally organized due to interactions with known structural abnormalities in other parts of the WMS brain (Galaburda & Bellugi, chap. 5; Reiss et al., chap. 4). From a developmental perspective, it was also important to examine whether the functional organization of brain systems linked to face processing in WMS might be similar to that found in normal brains at an earlier point in development. This result would indicate normal but delayed brain development. In contrast, it is also possible that WMS brains process this information in a different, perhaps unique, way.

In this study, we employed the event-related potential (ERP) technique to examine the organization of brain activity for face recognition, a spared cognitive function in WMS. We tested the hypothesis that the brain systems underlying face processing may be abnormally organized in WMS.

The Neural Basis of Abnormal Language Processing in WMS

In WMS, evidence from ERP studies of auditory language processing suggested abnormal patterns of cerebral specialization for language processing (Bellugi et al., 1999b; Bellugi, Lichtenberger, Mills, Galaburda, & Korenberg, 1999a; Mills, 1998; Neville, Mills, & Bellugi, 1994). Like face processing, auditory language comprehension and production have been shown to be remarkably spared in WMS adolescents and adults, in spite of the late onset of auditory language acquisition. Recent electrophysiological evidence (cited above) suggested that there were marked differences in the organization of language-relevant brain systems that might be unique to individuals with WMS. In normal adults and school-aged children, ERPs to closed class (i.e., grammatical function) words display a left-anterior asymmetry from at least 9 years of age. The presence of this asymmetry has been linked to performance on tests of comprehension of syntax (Neville, Coffey, Holcomb, & Tallal, 1993). Although WMS adolescents and adults have relatively spared grammatical abilities, most WMS subjects did not show the left-anterior asymmetry to closed class words. Additionally, WMS subjects showed an abnormally organized ERP response to processing semantic information in auditory sentences. Several ERP studies of normal adults and children have shown that a semantically anomalous word at the end of a sentence produces a robust negativity, called an N400, that has been linked to integration of word meaning (see Kutas & Hillyard, 1980). In adults, the visual N400 tends to be largest over posterior regions of the right hemisphere. However, in WMS subjects the N400 to semantic violations tended to be larger than normal and had a different distribution. In WMS, the N400 was larger over anterior than posterior regions and was larger from the left than the right hemisphere. In summary, the ERP studies of sentence processing described here suggest that the organization of neural systems that mediate different aspects of language, a spared cognitive function in WMS, is abnormally organized.

Face Processing and Other Spatial Abilities in WMS

Adolescents and adults with WMS have been shown to be quite adept at discriminating and learning to recognize unfamiliar faces. Behavioral studies suggest that most individuals with WMS are at, or close to, normal levels of performance on standardized tests of face processing, such as the Benton Test of Facial Recognition (Benton, Hamsher, Varney, & Spreen, 1983a), the Mooney Closure Test (Mooney, 1957), and the Warrington Recognition Memory Test (Warrington, 1984) (see Bellugi et al., 1999a; Bellugi et al., 1999b). This is in marked contrast to their impaired performance on tests of other spatial abilities. For example, most individuals with WMS are unable to match the angular orientation of two lines with lines in an array on the Benton Judgment of Line Orientation (Benton, Hamsher, Varney, & Spreen, 1983b), and perform very poorly on other form copying tasks such as the Test of Visual-Motor Integration (VMI; Beery, 1997), the block construction tasks in the Wechsler Intelligence Scale for Children—Revised (WISC; Wechsler, 1974) and in the Wechsler Adult Intelligence Scale—Revised (WAIS; Wechsler, 1981) (see Bellugi et al., chap. 1). Additionally, when asked to copy a line drawing of a house, WMS subjects tend to reproduce the local features, e.g., door, windows, chimney, but do not preserve the overall global configuration of the drawing (Bellugi et al., chap. 1). The tendency for WMS subjects to reproduce only the local elements in an array is also displayed in a hierarchical forms task (Bihrle, Bellugi, Delis, & Marks, 1989). For example, when asked to copy a large "Y" comprised of smaller "H"s, WMS subjects only produce the small "H"s, i.e., the local elements. This is of particular interest in relation to face-processing abilities that are generally thought to call on global or configural processing strategies in normal adults (Farah, Wilson, Drain, & Tanaka, 1998; Farah, Tanaka, & Drain, 1995; Tanaka & Farah, 1991; Diamond & Carey, 1986; Carey, Diamond, & Woods, 1980).

The hypothesis that upright faces are processed in a global or configural manner is supported by studies showing a disproportionate inversion effect for faces over other objects (Valentine, 1988; Diamond & Carey, 1986; Yin, 1969). The decrement in performance for recognition of inverted vs. upright faces is considerably larger than for other objects such as houses or cars. A series of recent studies by Farah et al. (1998) suggests that upright faces are recognized "holistically," whereas inverted faces and other types of objects are recognized by decomposition of their parts. One might predict that if WMS subjects show a bias for local processing, they would use similar strategies for processing upright and inverted faces. That is, they might not show an inversion effect. A preliminary study with WMS adults and adolescents supported this hypothesis (Rossen, Jones, Wang, & Klima, 1995). A recent study on children with WMS (ages 6 to 14 years) directly investigated the link between local/global strategies and performance on recognition of upright and inverted faces. In that study, most WMS children showed a preference for local processing on the hierarchical forms task. In contrast to the earlier study with adults, most WMS children showed a larger inversion effect than did normal age-matched controls (Jones, Hickok, & Lai, 1998). However, in that study, WMS children were presented with an example stimulus in the upright orientation and asked to find the matching face from an array of inverted stimuli. The mental rotation component, rather than the inversion of the stimuli, could have accounted for the increased decrement in performance. Moreover, in that study, behavioral scores on the matching task for upright and inverted faces were not correlated with scores on local/global processing. The results suggest that global processing of faces and hierarchical forms do not index the same processes.

Face-Specific Brain Mechanisms

The idea that there are brain systems specific to face recognition is supported by several lines of research. One line of evidence comes from brain-injured patients with prosopagnosia. These patients typically display an inability to recognize familiar faces without a concomitant decrement in other forms of object recognition. The lesions that produce the disorder are usually bilateral and extend along temporal and occipital cortical regions (Damasio, Tranel, & Damasio, 1990; Damasio, Damasio, & Van Hoesen, 1982). Some studies of patients with right-hemisphere lesions have described similar effects (Yin, 1970). A double dissociation exists in that other types of patients show preserved face-processing abilities with deficits in object recognition (Hécaen, Goldblum, Masure, & Ramier, 1974). Recently, Moscovitch, Winocur, and Behrmann (1997) described such a patient, CK, with normal face recognition but with object agnosia. CK performed as well as controls on tasks involving faces as long as they were upright and maintained the configurational properties of a face regardless of whether they were photographs, cartoons, or faces comprised of objects.

In normal adults, studies using brain-imaging techniques further support the hypothesis that there are specialized brain mechanisms within the occipito-temporal regions for face perception and recognition. A series of PET studies indicated increased regional blood flow within the fusiform gyrus in response to human faces (Sergent, Ohta, & MacDonald, 1992; Haxby et al., 1991; Haxby et al., 1994). Recent studies using fMRI have also shown activation of the fusiform gyrus in response to both passive viewing, and active matching tasks involving upright faces, but not to other types of visual stimuli including: non-face objects, scrambled faces, and inverted schematic (Mooney) faces, (Kanwisher, Tong, & Nakayama, 1998; Kanwisher, McDermott, & Chun, 1997; Clark, Maisog, & Haxby, 1997; McCarthy, Puce, Gore, & Allison, 1997; Clark et al., 1996; Puce, Allison, Gore, & McCarthy, 1995). Additionally, activation within this region was increased with selective attention to faces (Wojciulik, Kanwisher, & Driver, 1998).

Electrophysiological recordings made directly from occipito-temporal cortex in epileptic patients also showed activation to faces but not to other types of visual stimuli (Allison, McCarthy, Nobre, Puce, & Belger, 1994b; Allison, Puce, Spenser, & McCarthy, 1999; McCarthy, Puce, Belger, & Allison, 1999; Puce, Allison & McCarthy, 1999). A surface-negative potential at 200 msec, called the N200, was observed in response to faces but not scrambled faces, or pictures of cars, scrambled cars, or butterflies. Face-specific activity was observed in three regions: the ventral face area (lateral fusiform and adjacent inferior temporal gyri), the lateral face area (middle temporal gyri), and the anterior face area (anterior fusiform, cortex of the ventral-temporal pole and entorhinal cortex; Allison et al., 1999). The N200 was generated in the ventral and lateral face areas and was active during face perception but was not elicited by affective stimuli, diminished by habituation, affected by familiarity of the face, nor affected by semantic priming or face naming (Puce et al., 1999). Moreover, stimulation within face-specific regions produced an inability to name previously correctly identified faces (Allison et al., 1994a).

Face-specific ERPs have also been recorded from scalp electrodes (deHahn, Olivers, & Johnson, 1998; Bentin, Allison, Puce, Perez, & McCarthy, 1996; Botzel, Grusser, Haussler, & Naumann, 1989). A negative potential that peaked at 170 msec, called the N170, was elicited by faces and face components, especially eyes, but not by other types of visual stimuli (Bentin et al., 1996). Considering differences in the functional sensitivity of the N170 to eyes alone, and the depth and orientation of the fusiform where the N200 is generated, it is unlikely that the N170 and the subdural N200 reflect the same brain systems. Moreover, the N170 was maximal over right-posterior temporal regions and was, therefore, thought to be generated lateral to the fusiform region that generated the N200 (Bentin et al., 1996).

Preliminary research with WMS individuals also provided evidence consistent with the involvement of areas including the fusiform in face processing. In a study of WMS individuals (ages 10–20 years) using structural MRI, Jones et al. (1995) found that increased volume of gray matter in the inferior-posterior medial cortex, i.e., an area including the fusiform, was correlated with performance on the Benton Test of Facial Recognition. This finding raised the possibility that face perception and recognition may be normally organized in this population. However, the presence of structural abnormalities in posterior brain regions (Galaburda & Bellugi, chap. 5) raises the equally plausible hypothesis that the brain systems that underlie face processing in this population may be abnormally organized, or displaced anteriorly. This pattern might be reflected in a more anterior distribution of ERP effects, that is, increased activation, over the anatomically spared anterior regions.

Right Hemisphere Involvement in Face Processing

Several lines of evidence have suggested a greater involvement of the right than the left hemisphere in face processing, including: studies of patients with right-hemisphere lesions (de Renzi, 1986; Yin, 1970), epileptic patients who have undergone surgical callosectomy (Levy, Trevarthen, & Sperry, 1972), behavioral studies of normal subjects that have shown visual field preferences in face processing (e.g., Magnussen, Sunde, & Dyrnes, 1994; Schweinberger, Sommer, & Stiller, 1994; Schweinberger & Sommer, 1991; Sergent, 1986; Rhodes, 1985; Leehy, Carey, Diamond, and Cahn, 1978), brain imaging studies using PET and fMRI techniques that showed bilateral activation that was greater on the right side (Kanwisher et al., 1997; Kanwisher et al., 1998; McCarthy et al., 1997; Haxby et al., 1993; Sergent et al., 1992), and ERP studies that showed right-greater-than-left asymmetries in face-relevant components in adults (Alvarez, Mills, & Neville, 1999; deHahn et al., 1998; Bentin et al., 1996). A recent hemifield study using subdural recordings from epileptic patients suggested that the right hemisphere was better at processing information about upright faces, whereas the left hemisphere was better at processing information about inverted faces (McCarthy et al., 1999).

The present study was based on a recent ERP investigation of recognition for upright and inverted faces in normal adults (Alvarez et al., 1999). In that experiment, ERPs were recorded as subjects watched photographic pairs of upright or inverted faces presented sequentially on a computer monitor. The subject's task was to indicate whether the second face in the pair ("target") was the same or a different person as in the first photograph ("prime"). Results from normal adults showed marked differences in the timing and distribution of ERP effects linked to recognition of upright and inverted faces, and are consistent with other evidence suggesting that, in adults, nonidentical brain systems mediate processing of upright and inverted faces. Recognition of mismatched upright faces elicited a negativity at 320 msec and was most prominent over anterior regions of the right hemisphere (see also Barrett, Rugg, & Perrett, 1988). In contrast, ERPs to mismatched inverted faces were characterized by a positivity that occurred later (at 500 msec) and displayed a bilateral posterior distribution. These different patterns of brain activity are consistent with behavioral studies of adults suggesting that differences in processing upright and inverted faces may be associated with differences in processing configurational vs. featural information. Alvarez and Neville (1995) also used this paradigm to study the development of these brain systems in normal children at 9, 13, and 16 years of age. The results suggest that children, unlike adults, display a similar pattern of ERPs to upright and inverted faces. Moreover, the mature pattern of right-greater-than-left asymmetry to upright faces is not evident until the late teens. These data are consistent with behavioral research suggesting that children use a similar analysis strategy for both upright and inverted faces (Carey & Diamond, 1977).

Results

Behavioral Data

Normal adults were faster and more accurate than the WMS adults [main effect of group: reaction time, $F(1,1) = 10.28, p < .001$; accuracy, $F(1,1) = 21.69, p < .001$] (Figure 3.1). However, most of the WMS adults scored within the range of the normal adults. Examination of the accuracy data from individual subjects showed that for the upright faces 15 of the 18 WMS adults performed within the range of the normal adults (range for normal adults = 74–100%). For the inverted faces, 12 out of 18 WMS adults showed accuracy scores within the range of the normal adults (range for normal adults = 59–100%).

Both normal and WMS adults were faster and more accurate at recognizing upright than inverted faces [main effect of orientation: reaction time,[1] $F(1,35) = 11.67, p < .001$; accuracy, $F(1,39) = 114.89, p < .001$], and were faster and more accurate at correctly identifying matched than mismatched targets [main effect of condition: reaction time, $F(1,1) = 11.48, p < .001$; accuracy, $F(1,1) = 4.44, p < .05$].

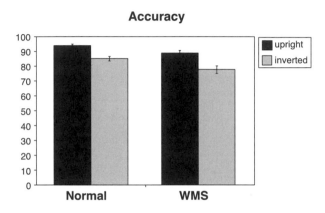

Figure 3.1
Error bars indicate the standard error of the mean. Top: Percent correct identification averaged across matched and mismatched targets. Bottom: Reaction time in msec for correct responses to matched and mismatched target faces.

Of particular importance was that the WMS and normal adults showed similar inversion effects. Relative to upright faces, inverted faces produced a 10% drop in accuracy and a 50 msec increase in reaction time for both the WMS and normal adults.

ERP Results

Results from a larger sample of normal controls on this paradigm are presented in Alvarez et al. (1999). The ERP patterns for the normal controls participating in this study are presented along with the data from the WMS subjects in the sections below. Any differences in the findings between the normal subjects in this sample and the previous study by Alvarez are noted in the corresponding analyses. For practical purposes, this chapter will emphasize group differences in responses to upright and inverted faces and matched vs. mismatched targets. The organization of the Results section is as follows: Each component is discussed separately in temporal order. The main effects for group differences are presented first. These effects are followed by main effects, and interactions with group, for orientation (upright vs. inverted), condition (match vs. mismatch), and distribution. Because ERPs between the two groups differed in amplitude, the data were normalized to assess true differences in distribution according to the formula recommended by McCarthy and Wood (1985).

Occipital sites are discussed separately due to differences in the latencies and morphology of the components over this area.

Primes: (i.e., the First Face in the Pair)   The morphology of the ERP components to the first face in the pair (prime) was similar to the targets, which are discussed in detail below (Figure 3.2).[2]

N100.   The first negative component peaked around 100 msec (N100). The latency of the N100 was later and the amplitude tended to be smaller in WMS subjects than normal controls [latency: group, $F(1,35) = 6.76$; amplitude: group, approached significance, $p < .10$]. Additionally, the amplitude of the N100 was larger from the left than the right hemisphere, but this effect was significant only for the normal controls [nor-

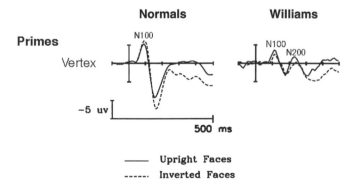

ERPs to Upright and Inverted Primes

Figure 3.2
ERPs to upright primes (solid) and inverted primes (dashed) are compared for normal subjects (left side) and WMS subjects (right side). Negative voltage is plotted up. Vertex refers to the electrode site (over the middle of the head) from which the ERPs shown in the figure were recorded.

malized amplitudes: hemisphere, $F(1,35) = 3.71$, $p = .06$; group × hemisphere, $p = .11$; for normal controls, hemisphere, $F(1,22) = 10.40$, $p < .001$; for WMS, n.s.]. The N100 was larger to inverted than upright faces, but again, only for the normal controls [amplitude: group × orientation, $F(1,35) = 8.79$, $p < .01$; amplitude for normal controls: orientation, $F(1,22) = 8.07$, $p < .01$; for WMS, n.s.].

P170.   The first positive component peaked around 170 msec (P170) for both normal and WMS subjects. The P170 was larger for normal than WMS adults [amplitude: group, $F(1,35) = 13.98$, $p < .001$]. Like the N100, the P170 was larger to inverted than upright faces, but only for the normal controls [amplitude: orientation, $F(1,35) = 4.66$, $p < .05$; group × orientation, $F(1,35) = 7.34$, $p < .01$; amplitude for normal controls, $F(1,22) = 14.71$, $p < .001$; WMS, n.s.].

N200.   There were no group differences or effects of orientation for the latency of the N200. The N200 response to both the prime and target stimuli (discussed below) was larger in WMS subjects than controls [amplitude: group, $F(1,35) = 29.39$, $p > .001$] (see Figures 3.2 and 3.3). The N200 was larger for upright than inverted faces for both groups [amplitude: orientation, $F(35) = 6.51$, $p < .05$].

N200 Peak Amplitude

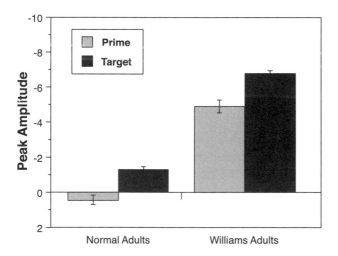

Figure 3.3
N200 amplitudes in μv for the first (prime) and second (target) faces presented within the pairs of stimuli. The N200 amplitudes are averaged across all cites anterior to the occiput. The results for normal adults are shown on the left and for WMS adults on the right. Results show N200 amplitudes for both primes and targets are dramatically larger for WMS than normal adults.

N300–500. The mean amplitude between 300 and 500 msec poststimulus onset was also examined for differences in ERPs to upright and inverted faces. For both normal and WMS adults, the mean amplitude between 300 and 500 was more negative for upright than inverted faces [$F(1,35) = 32.21$, $p < .001$]. Additionally, the N300–500 was larger over the left than the right hemisphere [mean amplitude: hemisphere, $F(1,35) = 5.04$, $p < .05$], and was larger over anterior than posterior regions [mean amplitude: electrode site, $F(3,105) = 49.54$, $p < .001$].

Targets: (i.e., Second Face in the Pair)   ERPs to the second face in the pair (target) were characterized by a series of negative and positive deflections in the following temporal order: A negativity at 200 msec, N200, and approximately 100 msec, N100; a positivity at 150 msec, P150; a negativity at 200 msec, N200, and 320 msec, N320; and a late positivity P500.

ERPs Anterior to the Occiput
N100.   The amplitude of the N100 was smaller, i.e., approximately half, for the WMS subjects than for the normal controls (mean; WMS = 5.7 μv, controls = 3.1 μv) [main effect of group: $F(3,117) = 6.92$, $p < .001$] (Figures 3.4 and 3.5). There was no main effect of group for peak latency.

For both groups, the N100 was larger and peaked later over anterior than posterior regions [main effect of electrode site: amplitude, $F(3,117) = 61.11$, $p < .001$, latency: $F(3,117) = 22.11$, $p < .001$]. And the N100 was larger and peaked later over the left than the right hemisphere [main effect of hemisphere: normalized amplitude, $F(1,39) = 5.52$, $p < .05$; latency, $F(1,39) = 4.60$, $p < .05$], especially over temporal and parietal regions, [normalized amplitude: hemisphere × electrode, $F(3,117) = 5.45$, $p < .01$]. However, the lateral effects for both latency and amplitude were significant for the normal controls but not the WMS subjects [latency: group × hemisphere, $F(1,39) = 4.40$, $p < .05$ (normal controls, $p < .01$; WMS, n.s.); group × hemisphere × electrode, $F(3,117) = 2.74$, $p < .05$ (normal controls, $p < .01$; WMS, n.s.); normalized amplitudes: group × hemisphere, approached significance, $F(1,39) = 2.89$, $p = .10$; group × orientation × hemisphere × electrode, $F(3,117) = 4.71$, $p < .01$]. Examination of the interactions with amplitude showed that the WMS subjects displayed a more symmetrical distribution of the N100.

For both groups, the N100 was smaller and peaked earlier to upright than inverted faces [main effect of orientation: amplitude, $F(1,39) = 5.08$, $p < .05$; latency, $F(1,39) = 12.07$, $p < .001$].

Previously, Alvarez et al. (1999) found that matched and mismatched targets elicited similar N100 responses. In the present study, there was a larger negativity to mismatched than matched targets [match/mismatch, $F(1,39) = 4.80$, $p < .05$]. Examination of an interaction with group, [normalized amplitude: group × match/mismatch × ori-

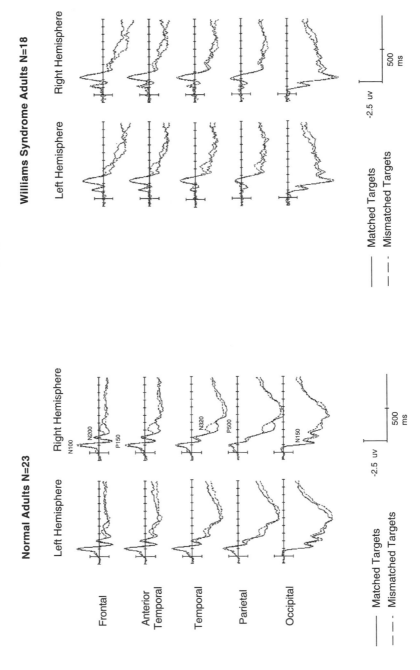

Figure 3.4
The solid line represents ERPs to targets that matched the preceding face. The dashed line represents ERPs to targets that differed (mismatch) from the preceding face.

Event-Related Potential Results for Inverted Faces Task

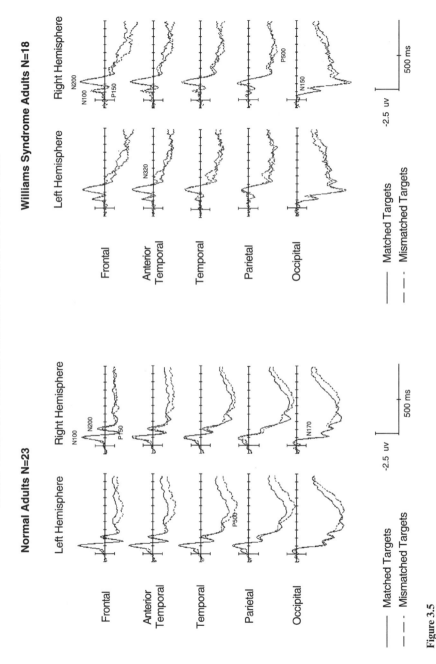

Figure 3.5
The solid line represents ERPs to targets that matched the preceding face. The dashed line represents ERPs to targets that differed (mismatch) from the preceding face.

entation × hemisphere, $F(1,39) = 6.37, p < .05$] showed that the match/mismatch effect approached significance for the WMS subjects, $p = .06$, but not the normal adults. Further examination of this interaction showed that for the WMS subjects the match/mismatch effect approached significance over the left hemisphere for upright faces, and over the right hemisphere for inverted faces.

P150.   Like the N100, the P150 was smaller, but also peaked earlier, in the WMS subjects than the normal controls [main effect of group: amplitude, $F(1,39) = 3.81, p < .05$; latency, $F(1,39) = 7.50, p < .01$].

Consistent with earlier findings (Alvarez et al., 1999), the P150 was earlier for upright than inverted faces for both groups [latency: $F(1,39) = 9.67, p < .001$]. In the Alvarez et al. (1999) study of normal adults, there were no other main effects or interactions for the P150. However, like the results from the N100, the WMS subjects, but not the normal controls, showed a significant difference in amplitude between the matched and mismatched targets [amplitude: group × match/mismatch: $F(1,39) = 12.70, p < .001$; main effect of match/mismatch for WMS subjects, $F(1,17) = 12.06, p < .001$; normal controls, n.s.].

N200.   The most striking difference in ERPs between the two groups was that the amplitude of the N200 was approximately six times larger in the WMS subjects (mean = -6.2, μv $SD = 3.4$) than in the normal controls (mean = -1.1, μv $SD = 3.9$) [amplitude: main effect of group: $F(1,39) = 35.90, p < .001$] (Figures 3.2, 3.3 and 3.4). The latency of the N200 was also 12 msec later in the WMS than in the normal adults [main effect of group: $F(1,39) = 6.54, p < .01$].

Like the previous results (Alvarez et al., 1999), the N200 was largest at frontal cites and peaked earliest over parietal cites [main effect of electrode: amplitude, $F(3,117) = 29.41, p < .001$; latency, $F(3,117) = 21.17, p < .001$.

The N200 was larger and earlier to upright than inverted faces [main effect of orientation: amplitude, $F(1,13) = 7.96, p < .01$, latency: $F(1,39) = 6.54, p < .01$]. But the amplitude effect was significant only for the WMS group [group × orientation, $F(1,39) = 4.95, p < .03$; orientation for WMS, $F(1,17) = 11.08, p < .01$; normal controls, n.s.].

Like the N100 and P150, the match/mismatch effect for N200 amplitude differed for WMS subjects and controls [group × match/mismatch, $F(1,39) = 10.04, p < .001$]. Although neither group showed a significant mismatch/match amplitude effect on the N200, the slope of the match/mismatch difference went in opposite directions. That is, for the WMS subjects, like the results from the N100, the N200 tended to be larger to mismatched than matched targets. The opposite trend was observed in the controls. Again, these data were consistent with the findings for the N100 and P150 showing earlier match/mismatch effects in the WMS subjects.

N320. The N320 was larger and peaked 30 msec later in the WMS than the control subjects [main effect of group: amplitude, $F(1,39) = 4.68$, $p < .04$; latency, $F(1,39) = 9.19$, $p < .001$]. However, the group differences were significant only over temporal and parietal regions [group × electrode: normalized amplitude, $F(3,117) = 3.46$, $p = .06$; latency, $F(3,117) = 5.09$, $p < .01$].

The N320 was largest over frontal regions [electrode site: amplitude, $F(3,117) = 52.45$, $p < .001$]. In the Alvarez et al. (1999) paper, the normal adults showed a right-hemisphere asymmetry over the anterior regions. In this study, the group × hemisphere × electrode interaction only approached significance [normalized amplitude, $F(3,11) = 2.43$, $p = .11$]. Because of the a priori hypothesis that WMS subjects may show abnormal asymmetries, we examined hemisphere effects separately for each group. Like the previous paper, the normal adults showed a right-hemisphere asymmetry over anterior regions [amplitude for normal adults: hemisphere × electrode site:, $F(3,66) = 5.52$, $p < .05$]. For the WMS subjects, the N320 tended to be larger from the left than the right but this effect did not reach statistical significance.

Like the N200, the N320 for both groups was larger and peaked earlier for upright than inverted faces [main effect of orientation: amplitude, $F(1,39) = 24.08$, $p < .001$; latency, $F(1,39) = 4.09$, $p < .05$].

Target faces that were different from the first face (mismatched targets) elicited a significantly larger and earlier N320 than did targets that matched the first face (Figure 3.3) [match/mismatch: amplitude, $F(1,39) = 34.22$, $p < .001$; latency, $F(1,39) = 14.55$, $p < .01$]. The match/mismatch difference was larger for the WMS than the normal adults [amplitude: group × match/mismatch: $F(1,39) = 9.49$, $p < .001$]. Moreover, the lateral distribution of the match/mismatch difference was opposite in the two groups, [normalized amplitude, group × match/mismatch × hemisphere: $F(1,39) = 4.13$, $p < .05$]. That is, the match/mismatch difference tended to be larger from the right than the left for normal controls, but larger from the left than the right in WMS subjects. Both of these trends only approached significance.

Upright and inverted faces elicited different match/mismatch patterns [amplitude: orientation × condition, $F(1,39) = 13.56$, $p < .001$]. However, this pattern differed for the normals and WMS subjects [normalized amplitude: group × orientation × match/mismatch × electrode, $F(3,117) = 3.95$, $p < .05$]. As in Alvarez et al. (1999), normal adults displayed a larger N320 to the mismatched than the matched targets for upright, but not inverted, faces [amplitude for normal adults: orientation × match/mismatch, $F(1,22) = 5.22$, $p < .03$; upright faces: match/mismatch, $F(1,22) = 11.86$, $p < .001$; inverted faces, n.s.]. In contrast, the WMS subjects displayed an N320 match/mismatch effect for both upright and inverted faces [amplitude for WMS: upright faces: match/mismatch, $F(1,17) = 41.89$, $p < .001$; inverted faces: match/mismatch, $F(1,17) = 8.68, p < .01$]. However, even in the WMS group, the effect was attenuated for the inverted faces [amplitude for WMS: orientation × match/mismatch, $F(1,17) = 8.14, p < .01$].

P500.   A positive slow-wave component that peaked around 500 msec, the P500, was larger for controls than WMS subjects over temporal and parietal regions [normalized mean area: group × electrode, $F(3,117) = 20.03, p < .001$. Examination of this interaction showed that although the P500 was larger over posterior than anterior regions for both groups [normalized mean area: electrode site, $F(3,117) = 72.03, p < .001$], the posterior distribution appeared to be more pronounced in the normal controls [mean area for normal controls: electrode site: $F(3,66) = 65.63, p < .001$; mean area for WMS, electrode site $F(3,51) = 8.68, p < .01$; see Figures 3.4 and 3.5].

As in the previous study (Alvarez et al., 1999), the normal adults displayed a larger P500 to mismatched than matched targets, for the inverted but not the upright faces (Figure 3.5) [mean area for normal adults: orientation × match/mismatch, $F(1,22) = 9.68, p < .01$; inverted, match/mismatch, $F(1,22) = 14.41, p < .001$; upright, match/mismatch, n.s.]. In contrast, the WMS subjects did not show a significant P500 match/mismatch effect for either the upright or inverted faces [mean area: group × match/mismatch, $F(1,39) = 5.45, p < .05$; mean area for WMS: match/mismatch, n.s.].

ERPs over Occipital Regions
P100.   The first positive component peaked at 116 msec. There were no group differences in the latency of the P100. Like the anterior N100, the occipital P100 appeared to be smaller in the WMS subjects than controls, but the difference did not reach significant levels.

N150.   The first negative component peaked at approximately 150 msec for both groups. In contrast to the anterior P150, the N150 was larger in the WMS than normal adults [group, amplitude, $F(1,39) = 7.24, p < .01$]. However, like the anterior P150, the WMS subjects but not the normal controls showed a match/mismatch effect, suggesting earlier recognition processes in the WMS subjects [group × match/mismatch, amplitude, $F(1,39) = 15.42, p < .001$; WMS, match/mismatch, amplitude, $F(1,17) = 6.86, p < .02$].

N200.   The second negative component peaked earlier for the normal controls (257 msec) than for the WMS subjects (280 msec) [latency: group, $F(1,39) = 10.56, p < .001$]. In contrast to the anterior N200, there were no group differences in the amplitude of the N200 over the occiput. The mismatched faces elicited a larger N200 than did the matched faces [amplitude: match/mismatch, [$F(1,39) = 7.03$].

N320.   Like the occipital N200, the N320 tended to be earlier for the normal controls (382 msec) than for the WMS subjects (393 msec) [latency: group, $F(1,39) = 3.75$, $p = .06$, n.s.). The mean amplitude of the N320 was larger for mismatched than matched targets [mean area: match/mismatch, $F(1,39) = 3.88$, $p = .06$]. However, unlike the anterior N320, this effect did not interact with orientation. The match/mismatch effect tended to be larger from the right than the left hemisphere for the normal controls and tended to be larger from the left than the right for the WMS subjects [normalized mean area: group × hemisphere, $F(1,39) = 6.30$, $p < .05$]. However, the effect of hemisphere was not significant for either group alone.

P500.   Like the anterior cites, the P500 was larger to mismatched than matched targets, only for inverted faces, and only for the normal controls [mean area: group × match/mismatch, $F(1,39) = 4.32$, $p < .05$; orientation × match/mismatch; $F(1,39) = 5.37$, $p < .05$; inverted faces: group × match/mismatch, $F(1,39) = 5.61$, $p < .05$]. The P500 match/mismatch effect was larger over the left than the right hemisphere for normal controls, but not for WMS subjects [mean area: group × hemisphere, $F(1,39) = 5.37$, $p < .05$].

Correlations with Benton Scores and ERP and Task Performance Scores in WMS   Only the WMS subjects had scores for the Benton Test of Facial Recognition (Benton et al., 1983a, b; see Table 3.1). Therefore, the following correlations and other statistical treatments apply only to the WMS subjects.

BENTON SCORES AND ACCURACY ON ERP TASK.   The WMS subjects with higher Benton Test of Facial Recognition scores tended to be more accurate on the match/mismatch task [Spearman, $r = 43$, $p = .07$; Pearson, $r = .45$, $p < .05$].

Table 3.1
Characteristics of Subjects with Williams Syndrome in Comparison to Normal Performance Based on Standardized Scores

	Age (years)	FSIQ	Benton	PPVT
Williams Subjects				
mean	25	61	22	62
range	18–38	51–76	17–26	33–79
standard deviation	5.9	16.9	2.9	12.22
Normal Performance				
standardized mean		100	22	100
standard deviation		15	3	15

FSIQ = Full scale IQ from Weschler adult intelligence scale.
BENTON = Benton Face Recognition Test.
PPVT = Peabody Picture Vocabulary Test.

BENTON SCORES AND N200 AMPLITUDE.   Because the N200 was dramatically larger in WMS than normal adults, we were particularly interested in its functional significance. WMS subjects with larger amplitude N200 components tended to score higher on the Benton Test of Facial Recognition [Spearman, $r = .51$, $p < .05$; Pearson, $r = .38$, $p = .10$; see Figure 3.6, top]. Because the Pearson correlation only approached significance, we further examined the relationship between the Benton scores and the N200 amplitude. Subjects were divided into two groups based on their scores on the short form of the Benton Test of Facial Recognition. Those who scored above 23 were designated as the high group: i.e., high Benton group, mean = 24.3, range 23 to 26; and low Benton group, mean = 19.3, range 17 to 22. The high Benton group had larger N200 amplitudes than did the low Benton group [for WMS group: $F(1,16) = 6.61$, $p < .05$].

BENTON SCORES AND N320 MATCH/MISMATCH LATENCY FOR UPRIGHT FACES.   We predicted that WMS subjects who scored higher on the Benton might also show earlier ERP effects of face recognition. In the original study, the match/mismatch effect for face recognition occurred on the N320 for upright faces. However, neither the amplitude nor the latency of the N320 match/mismatch effect was correlated with scores on the Benton. In contrast, for the WMS subjects the latency of the N320 match/mismatch effect was positively correlated with reaction time on the ERP task [Spearman, $r = .54$, $p < .05$; Pearson, $r = .46$, $p < .05$; ANOVA for WMS group: $F(1,16) = 7.07$, $p < .05$; see Figure 3.6, bottom].

BENTON AND P500 MATCH/MISMATCH EFFECT FOR INVERTED FACES.   Earlier studies using this paradigm showed that the P500 match/mismatch effect for inverted faces develops with increasing age and proficiency. In the present study, the WMS subjects did not show this effect. Therefore, we examined whether the WMS subjects who scored high on the Benton and/or high on accuracy on the match/mismatch task would show the P500 effect for inverted faces. There were no correlations or other significant differences based on the high Benton vs. low Benton groups described above.

Discussion

ERP Indices of Face Perception

In individuals with WMS, the morphology of the first 200 msec of the ERP waveform in response to faces for both primes and target stimuli was strikingly different from normal. For primes, the N100 and P170 components were smaller for WMS than normal adults. In contrast, the WMS adults displayed an N200 to primes that was absent or attenuated in the ERPs to primes from normal adults. For target stimuli, the ampli-

ERP Effects of High and Low Scores on Benton Faces

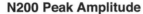

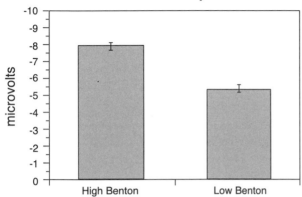

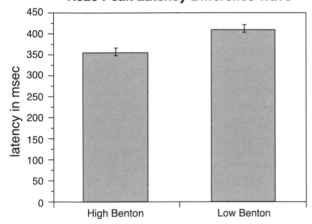

Figure 3.6
Differences in ERPs for WMS subjects who scored high vs. low on the Benton Facial-Recognition Task. The group differences were based on a median split of the data. The top half of the figure shows a larger amplitude N200 response by WMS subjects who scored in the High Benton group. The bottom half of the figure shows that subjects who scored in the High Benton group tended to have an earlier N320-peak latency for the mismatch minus mismatch difference wave.

tude of the N100 in WMS subjects was approximately half the amplitude of the N100 in normal adults. In contrast, the amplitude of the N200 to targets was more than twice the size of the N200 in normal adults. These differences were not subtle, that is, they were larger than two standard deviations of the mean for the normal subjects. This ERP pattern, a small N100 and large N200, was observed in all of the adult subjects with WMS reported here, as well as in all children with WMS we have tested (unpublished data). We have not observed these ERP patterns in normal adults, children, or infants at any age, nor in any of the other populations (i.e., Down syndrome, language impaired children, children with early left- or right-hemisphere brain injury) we have studied. Importantly, these ERP patterns were not observed in two subjects who had a clinical diagnosis of WMS but who did not have the genetic deletion based on the florescence in situ hybridization (FISH) test (not included in this sample). However, to the extent that ERPs index information about brain function, we would expect to find variables that modulate the amplitude and latency of these components in other populations who share specific neurological and neurocognitive characteristics in common with WMS. It is also possible that these effects are linked to subtle structural abnormalities, e.g., abnormal folding or orientation of sulci in the areas generating these components, which may be present in all individuals with WMS (see Galaburda & Bellugi, chap. 5, for a discussion of abnormal configuration of gyri in WMS). Another consideration is that the amplitude of the N200 was correlated with performance on the Benton Test of Facial Recognition. This is of particular interest because larger volumetric measures of the inferior-posterior medial cortex revealed in MRI analyses were also correlated with performance on the Benton Test of Facial Recognition in WMS subjects (Jones et al., 1995).

We are currently conducting a study of black and white photographs of upright and inverted cars to determine whether the abnormal N100/N200 complex in WMS is specific to face processing. Preliminary results from 10 normal adults and 10 adults with WMS are shown in the right side of Figure 3.7. Based on visual inspection of the data from individual subjects, there were two main findings. First, the ERP patterns observed for faces, i.e., small N100/larger N200 pattern for WMS, and larger N100/ smaller N200 pattern for normal controls were also present to cars (Mills, St. George, & Zangl, unpublished data). This finding could be consistent with the hypothesis that the abnormal N100/N200 pattern indexes activity related to general object perception and might be linked to structural abnormalities in the temporo-occipital regions including the fusiform gyrus. However, the ERP differences between WMS and control subjects were more pronounced for faces than for cars. Second, for both normal controls and WMS subjects, ERPs to cars differed from ERPs to faces. At first glance, it appeared that the ERPs were just larger to faces than to cars. However, the amplitude

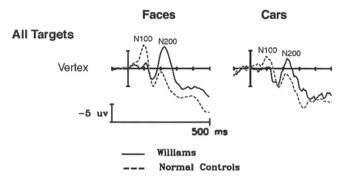

ERPs to Faces and Cars for Normal and WMS Adults

Figure 3.7
ERPs for WMS (solid lines) subject are directly compared with normal subjects (dashed lines) for faces on the left side of the figure and for cars on the right side of the figure. ERPs to cars were recorded from an additional 10 normal adults and 10 adults with WMS (ages 18 to 24). The data for faces were from the 23 normal and 18 WMS subjects described in this study.

differences were more complex. For WMS subjects, the N100 was approximately the same size for faces and cars, but the amplitude of the N200 was markedly reduced for cars. This pattern of results is consistent with the hypothesis that the amplitude of the N200 may be linked to increased attention to faces in WMS. For normal controls, the N100 was larger to faces than to cars, whereas the N200 was similar in amplitude to faces and cars. Additionally, both the anterior-posterior and lateral distributions of the N100 and N200 differed for cars and faces for WMS and normal subjects. This finding is important because it provides further evidence that faces and objects are mediated by non-identical neural systems. Although the abnormal N100/N200 complex in WMS may not be specific to faces, it appeared to be different for faces as compared to non-face stimuli.

In studies of normal visual processing, the N100 and N200 components have been linked to perceptual and attentional rather than recognition processes per se (Mangun & Hillyard, 1991). In normal adults, studies of non-face visual stimuli have shown that the amplitude of the N100 increases with attention, and is sensitive to the physical parameters of the visual stimuli, i.e., it increases with increased stimulus intensity, and is probably generated in extrastriate visual cortex (e.g., Mangun, Hillyard, & Luck, 1993). The N200 has been linked with discrimination, categorization, and feature identification (Polich, Ellerson, & Cohen, 1996; Harter, Ainne, & Schroeder, 1984; Hillyard & Kutas, 1983).

In the present study, match/mismatch effects, that is, larger amplitude ERPs to the mismatched targets, were observed on the N100, P150, and N200 in subjects with WMS but not in the normal adult controls. Research with normal adults has shown that the amplitudes of both the N100 and N200 components are modulated by attentional effects (see Hillyard, Mangun, Woldorff, & Luck, 1995 for a review). Moreover, attention to faces has been shown to lead to increased activity in the fusiform, i.e., the area linked to face perception (Wojciulik et al., 1998). Anecdotal evidence from individuals with WMS shows increased interest and fixation on human faces, especially the eyes (Bellugi et al., chap. 1). Therefore, we propose that the earlier match/mismatch effect in WMS may be due to increased attention to faces in WMS.

It is unlikely that the N200 observed in the present study is the same N200 response observed in subdural recordings (Allison et al., 1994a; Allison et al., 1994b). The N200 observed here had an anterior distribution. As noted by Bentin et al. (1996), the orientation of the neurons producing a surface negative potential over the fusiform region would not produce a negative ERP over more superior scalp. It is also equally unlikely that the N200 observed here is the same component as the N170 described by Bentin, which was specific to faces and face components (Bentin et al., 1996). The N200 in the present study and the N170 also displayed different distribution. The N170 was maximal over occipito-temporal regions, T5/T6 (not recorded here), vs. the anterior distribution of the N200. However, it is possible that the occipital N150 observed here may index the same systems as the occipito-temporal N170. In the present study, the occipital N150 was larger in WMS than normal adults. This is consistent with the hypothesis that WMS individuals have increased neural activity to faces. Further research is needed to test this hypothesis.

ERP Patterns Linked to Recognition

On the ERP face-recognition task, normal adults were faster and more accurate than the subjects with WMS. However, both groups displayed similar behavioral inversion effects. That is, both groups were 10% less accurate and 50 msec slower to recognize inverted than upright faces. Unlike the normal adults, the WMS subjects did not show marked differences in the morphology, latency and distribution of the match/mismatch effect to upright and inverted faces. For upright faces, both the normal adults and adults with WMS showed a larger N320 component to the mismatched targets. This effect displayed an anterior distribution and was larger from the right than the left hemisphere in the normal adults. In the WMS subjects, the N320 effect also displayed an anterior distribution but tended to be larger from the left than the right. For inverted faces, the normal adults did not show an N320 effect. Rather, the mismatched inverted faces elicited a positive component, which peaked later around 500 msec, displayed a posterior distribution and was symmetrical. In contrast, the WMS subjects displayed an N320 effect that was smaller for inverted than upright faces, but displayed the same anterior-posterior and lateral distributions for upright and inverted faces. That is, the orientation of the stimuli modulated the amplitude of the effect, but did not provide evidence of distinct neural systems. These findings are consistent with earlier behavioral studies suggesting that in individuals with WMS, similar brain systems mediate recognition of upright and inverted faces (Rossen et al., 1995).

Examination of developmental data from an experiment using the same paradigm in normal 9-, 13-, 16-, 18-, and 22+-year-olds revealed that for the WMS subjects, behavioral performance on the face-recognition task was similar in accuracy and reaction times to the average performance of 13-year-old normal children (Alvarez & Neville, 1995). Similar to the WMS subjects, the ERP effects for normal 13-year-olds displayed an N320 effect that was the same amplitude for upright and inverted faces and was larger over the left than the right hemisphere. In contrast, the amplitudes of the N100 and N200 were dramatically different in WMS adults and normal 13-year-olds. Like normal adults, the normal 13-year-olds showed larger N100 than N200 components to faces. These results suggested that in contrast to the brain systems that mediate face *perception,* which are abnormal in WMS, the brain systems that mediate face *recognition* might be normally organized but developmentally delayed.

Conclusion

Based on the findings presented here, we offer the following conclusions: ERP patterns that index face *recognition,* that is, the N320 match/mismatch effect, suggest that adults with WMS, like normal children, do not employ markedly different brain systems for recognizing upright and inverted faces, as do normal adults. Additionally, we propose that the early match/mismatch effects on the N100, P150, and N200 components, which were not observed in the normal controls, might be linked to increased attention to faces in WMS and, in part, may arise from and mediate the remarkably spared function in this population. In contrast, abnormalities in the early ERP patterns that index face *perception* may be specific to WMS. Because the small N100/large N200 complex to faces was observed in all WMS subjects, including children with WMS whose data were not reported here, and has not been observed in any of the other clinical populations we have tested, nor in normal development at any age between 3 and 35 years, we believe the abnormal N100/N200 complex might be an electrophysiological marker for abnormal face perception in WMS. We will further evaluate whether these effects are specific to faces in our ongoing electrophysiological and behavioral studies of object recognition. Although sparing of the ventral-visual stream is likely to be associated with spared face-recognition abilities in this population (Galaburda & Bellugi, chap. 6 Atkinson et al., 1997), the reliability of this abnormal N100/N200 complex suggests that it may be linked to subtle structural abnormalities, for example, abnormal orientation of specific sulci, which are common among all individuals with WMS. In our continuing studies, we plan to examine whether the variability in the amplitudes and scalp distributions of these components can be linked to variability in neurological and genetic profiles of individuals with WMS.

Methods

Subjects

Subjects included 18 adults (18–38 yr, mean = 25 yr; 9 females) with WMS and 23 normal adults (18–38 yr, mean = 24 yr; 13 females). All but three of the WMS subjects were right handed as determined by handedness and medical questionnaires. All subjects with WMS were diagnosed clinically by a medical geneticist prior to induction into the study through genetic probes and medical/genetic records. Subjects were part of the Program Project "Williams Syndrome: Bridging Cognition and Gene," and concurrently took part in neurocognitive, neuromorphological, electrophysiological, and molecular genetic probes (see Preface and Bellugi et al., chap. 1). Subjects were excluded from the study if they had a history of concurrent medical conditions not typically associated with WMS, particularly those with confounding medical or neurological consequences. All clinical diagnoses were confirmed by trained researchers using the Williams Syndrome Diagnostic Scoresheet, a screening measure developed by the medical advisory board of the Williams Syndrome Association.

Additional information for the WMS subjects is provided in Table 3.1. Normal adults were all native monolingual speakers of English and were right handed as determined by the Edinburgh Handedness Assessment. All subjects had normal or corrected-to-normal vision.

Stimuli

The stimuli were the same as described in Alvarez et al., (1999). The stimuli consisted of 38 pairs of digitized black and white photographs of adult faces (half female) displayed on a video monitor. Each model displayed a neutral facial expression. To control for differences in hairstyle, all of the models were wearing the same gender-appropriate wig. There were two variations of physiognomy (same or different person), and orientation (right-side-up or upside-down, see Figure 3.8). On one-half of the trials, both faces in a

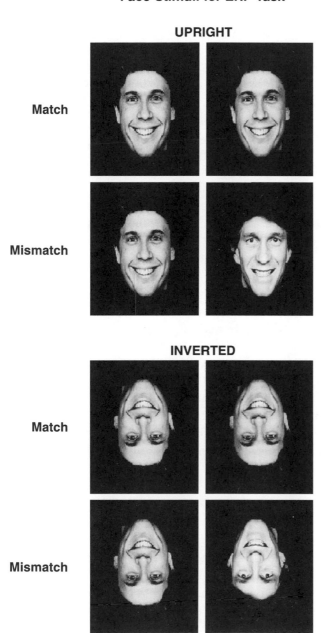

Figure 3.8
Sample stimuli for primes (left column) and targets (right column) for all four conditions (top: upright matched and upright mismatched; bottom: inverted matched and inverted mismatched).

pair were the same person; on the other half, the photographs were of different people (same gender). In the condition where the faces were of the same person, two different photographs were used. Half of the images in each condition were presented right-side up and half were upside-down. When different faces within a pair were presented, complexion and outer contour shape of the faces were similar.

Procedure

The experiment was conducted in a sound attenuated chamber. The video monitor was placed 57 in. from the bridge of the subject's nose. At the beginning of each trial, the subjects fixated on a small cross in the center of the screen. The subjects initiated each trial by pressing a button. Trials consisted of the sequential presentation of two faces. Each face was shown for 1500 msec with an inter-stimulus interval (ISI) of 1000 msec between faces (see Figure 3.8). The subject was instructed to press a button labeled either "yes" or "no" as quickly as possible to indicate whether the second face matched (yes—was the same person) or did not match (no—different person) the first face. Fifteen practice trials were given before the experiment began.

ERP Recording

The electroencephalogram (EEG) was recorded using tin electrodes (Electro-cap International) from 14 sites over left and right frontal, (Fp1/Fp2, F7/F8), anterior temporal (one-half the distance between F7/F8 and T3/T4), temporal (33% of the distance from T3/T4 to C3/C4), left and right parietal (50% of the distance between T3/T4 and P3/P4), midline (Cz, Pz), and occipital regions (O1/O2). Additionally, the electrooculogram from over (Fp1) and under the left eye was recorded to monitor blinks and vertical eye movements and from the right outer canthus to monitor horizontal eye movements. Impedances were maintained below 5 kΩ. All electrodes were referenced to linked mastoids. The EEG was filtered with a bandpass of .01 to 100 Hz.

Data Analysis

Behavioral Data

Accuracy scores and reaction times were calculated for each condition: Upright faces (matched and mismatched), and inverted faces (matched and mismatched). Responses were classified as correct for those trials on which the subject pressed the appropriate button within 200–3000 msec after the onset of the target stimulus (i.e., pressed the "Yes" button when the prime and target were the same person, or the "No" button when the prime and target were different faces). Reaction times were calculated as the latency from the onset of the target stimulus to the button press for a correct response.

Event-Related Potential Data

ARTIFACT REJECTION.   Artifact rejection was conducted off-line using a custom computer program. Criteria for rejection of trials containing eye blinks, horizontal eye movement, muscle movement, or amplifier blocking were set for each subject individually based on visual inspection of the data on a trial-by-trial basis. ERPs for correct responses were then averaged separately for primes and targets. For prime stimuli, the ERPs were averaged separately according to orientation (upright or inverted). For target stimuli, the ERPs were averaged separately according to the type of stimulus pair presented (i.e., upright matched, upright mismatched, inverted matched, inverted mismatched). ERP component amplitudes were quantified with reference to a 100 msec prestimulus baseline. Peak latencies and amplitudes (for the maximum negative or positive voltage in a specified time window) were measured for all components showing a clear peak. Mean area measurements (the mean voltage in a specified time window) were taken for components without clear peaks, i.e., the occipital N320, and the anterior and occipital P500 to the target stimuli.

COMPONENT DEFINITIONS AND MEASUREMENTS.   All measurements were relative to a 100 msec prestimulus baseline. For the prime stimuli, the first negative component peaked around 100 msec, called the N100, and was defined as the most negative peak occurring between 50 and 150 msec after stimulus onset. The first positive component peaked at approximately 170 msec, called the P170, and was defined as the most positive peak between 100 and 250 msec. The next negative peak observed, referred to as the N200, was measured within a window of 150–275 msec poststimulus onset. The N300–500 was defined as the mean amplitude between 300 and 500 msec.

For target stimuli, at electrodes anterior to the occiput, the first component was negative-going and peaked around 100 msec, called the N100. The N100 was defined as the most negative peak occurring between 50 and 150 msec poststimulus onset. The next component, called the P150, was positive and peaked at approximately 150 msec. The P150 was defined as the most positive peak between 100 and 200 msec poststimulus onset. A second negative component observed at approximately 200 msec, called the N200, was measured within a window of 150–275 msec poststimulus onset. A third negative component, called the N320, peaked at approximately 320 msec, and was measured within a window of 250–400 msec poststimulus onset. Finally, a late, positive-going waveform, called the P500, was measured between 400 and 800 msec poststimulus onset.

Over the left and right occipital sites, the first peak was a positive component that peaked at approximately 100 msec, called the P100. The P100 was defined as the most positive peak occurring between 50 and 150 msec (P100). Following the P100, a negative component, called the N100, was measured within a window of 100–225 msec post-stimulus onset. The second negative peak, called the N200, was measured between 200 and 325 msec after stimulus onset. The third negative peak over the occipital regions was observed between 325 and 450 msec poststimulus onset, called the N320. Finally, the P500 was also observed over the occiput and was measured within the same window at more anterior electrodes, 400–800 msec poststimulus onset.

NORMALIZATION PROCEDURES.   To examine the group differences in the distribution of ERP effects, the data were normalized according to the procedures outlined by Mc-Carthy and Wood (1985). Analyses including main effects and interactions with hemisphere and electrode site are reported for the normalized amplitudes.

DATA ANALYSIS.   Statistical analyses were conducted for each of the components separately. The design employed a mixed-model ANOVA using the BMDP 4V program with Geisser and Greenhouse corrections for repeated measures (Geisser & Greenhouse, 1959). For the prime stimuli, the ANOVA included two levels of group (normal and WMS), two levels of orientation (upright and inverted), two levels of hemisphere (left and right), and four levels of electrode (frontal, anterior temporal, temporal and parietal). For the target stimuli, the ANOVAs were performed with the levels described above plus two levels of condition (matched and mismatched). Because the morphology (i.e., presence or absence of specific peaks) of the waveforms differed over occipital and more anterior sites, separate ANOVAs were conducted for occipital sites and for sites anterior to the occiput. The ANOVAs for the occipital measures included two levels of group (normal and WMS), two levels of orientation (upright and inverted), two levels of condition (match, mismatch), and two levels of hemisphere (left and right). When it was necessary to explore significant effects or interactions, appropriate simple effects tests were used for a priori hypotheses; post hoc comparisons were conducted using Tukey's HSD tests (Tukey, 1977).

Notes

The research was supported by grants from the National Institute of Child Health and Human Development (P01 HD33113 to U. Bellugi), National Institute of Deafness and Communication Disorders (P50 DC01289 to E. Bates), and the National Institute of Neurological Disorders and Strokes (P50 NS22343 to E. Bates). The authors are grateful to the regional and national Williams Syndrome Associations and all the individuals with Williams syndrome who helped make these studies possible. We would like to thank Marta Kutas, Johnathan King, and Steve Hillyard for their valuable feedback on interpretation of the data, and Ed Klima for his insightful comments on earlier versions of this paper. We would also like to thank Chantel Prat and Renate Zangl for their help in data collection, and Wendy Jones and Zona Lai for providing the scores on the Benton Test of Facial Recognition.

1. Due to computer problems, reaction time data were lost for four of the normal adults.

2. Due to a technical problem, ERPs to the primes are available for 14 of the 18 adults with WMS.

Illustrations and quotes not to be used without written permission from the author. Copyright Dr. Debra L. Mills, La Jolla, CA.

References

Allison, T., Ginter, H., McCarthy, G., Nobre, A. C., Puce, A., Luby, M., & Spencer, D. D. (1994a). Face recognition in human extrastriate cortex. *Journal of Neurophysiology, 71,* 821–825.

Allison, T., McCarthy, G., Nobre, A., Puce, A., & Belger, A. (1994b). Human extrastriate visual cortex and the perception of faces, words, numbers, and colors. Special Issue: Object recognition and the temporal lobes. *Cerebral Cortex, 4,* 544–554.

Allison, T., Puce, A., Spencer, D. D., & McCarthy, G. (1999). Electrophysiological studies of human face perception. I: Potentials generated in occipitotemporal cortex by face and non-face stimuli. *Cerebral Cortex, 9,* 415–430.

Alvarez, T. D., Mills, D., & Neville, H. J. (1999). Different neural mechanisms for upright and inverted face recognition: Electrophysiological evidence [*Tech. Rep.* #9905]. La Jolla, University of California at San Diego, Center for Research in Language.

Alvarez, T. D., & Neville, H. J. (1995). The development of face recognition continues into adulthood: An ERP study. *Neuroscience Abstracts, 21,* 2086.

Atkinson, J., King, J., Braddick, O., Nokes, L., Anker, S., & Braddick, F. (1997). A specific deficit of dorsal stream function in Williams syndrome. *NeuroReport, 8,* 1919–1922.

Beery, K. E. (1997). *The Beery-Buktenica developmental test of visual-motor integration* (Fourth Edition, Revised). Parsippany, NJ: Modern Curriculum Press.

Barrett, S. E., Rugg, M. D., & Perrett, D. I. (1988). Event-related potentials and the matching of familiar and unfamiliar faces. *Neuropsychologia, 26,* 105–117.

Bellugi, U., Lichtenberger, L., Jones, W., Lai, Z., & St. George, M. (chap. 1). The neurocognitive profile of Williams Syndrome: A complex pattern of strengths and weaknesses.

Bellugi, U., Lichtenberger, L., Mills, D., Galaburda, A., & Korenberg, J. (1999a). Bridging cognition, brain and molecular genetics: Evidence from Williams syndrome. *Trends in Neurosciences, 22,* 197–207.

Bellugi, U., Mills, D., Jernigan, T., Hickok, G., & Galaburda, A. (1999b). Linking cognition, brain structure and brain function in Williams syndrome. In H. Tager-Flusberg (Ed.), *Neurodevelopmental disorders: Contributions to a new framework from the cognitive neurosciences* (pp. 111–136). Cambridge, MA: MIT Press.

Bentin, S., Allison, T., Puce, A., Perez, E., & McCarthy, G. (1996). Electrophysiological studies of face perception in humans. *Journal of Cognitive Neuroscience, 8,* 551–565.

Benton, A. L., Hamsher, K. de S., Varney, N. R., & Spreen, O. (1983a). *Benton test of facial recognition.* New York, NY: Oxford University Press.

Benton, A. L., Hamsher, K. de S., Varney, N. R., & Spreen, O. (1983b). *Benton judgment of line orientation, form H.* New York, NY: Oxford University Press.

Bihrle, A. M., Bellugi, U., Delis, D., & Marks, S. (1989). Seeing either the forest or the trees: Dissociation in visuospatial processing. *Brain and Cognition, 11,* 37–49.

Botzel, K., Grusser, O. J., Haussler, B., & Naumann, A. (1989). The search for face-specific evoked potentials. In E. Basar & T. H. Bullock (Eds.), *Springer series in brain dynamics 2* (pp. 449–467). Berlin: Springer-Verlag.

Carey, S., & Diamond, R. (1977). From piecemeal to configurational representation of faces. *Science, 195,* 312–314.

Carey, S., Diamond, R., & Woods, B. (1980). Development of face recognition: A maturational component? *Developmental Psychology, 16,* 257–269.

Clark, V. P., Keil, K., Maisog, J. M., Courtney, S., Ungerleider, L. G., & Haxby, J. V. (1996). Functional magnetic resonance imaging of human visual cortex during face matching: A comparison with positron emission tomography. *Neuroimage, 4,* 1–15.

Clark, V. P., Maisog, J. M., & Haxby J. V. (1997). fMRI studies of visual perception and recognition using a randomized stimulus design. *Society for Neuroscience Abstracts, 23,* 301.

Damasio, A. R., Damasio, H., & Van Hoesen, G. W. (1982). Prosopagnosia: Anatomic basis and behavioral mechanisms. *Neurology, 32,* 331–341.

Damasio, A. R., Tranel, D., & Damasio, H. (1990). Face agnosia and the neural substrates of memory. *Annual Review of Neuroscience, 13,* 89–109.

deHahn, M., Olivers, A., & Johnson, M. H. (1998). Electrophysiological correlates of face processing by adults and 6-month-old infants. *Cognitive Neuroscience Society 1998 Annual Meeting Abstract Program* 36.

de Renzi, E. (1986). Prosopagnosia in two patients with CT scan evidence of damage confined to the right hemisphere. *Neuropsychologia, 24,* 385–389.

Diamond, R., & Carey, S. (1986). Why faces are and are not special: An effect of expertise. *Journal of Experimental Psychology: General, 115,* 107–117.

Farah, M. J., Tanaka, J. W., & Drain, H. M. (1995). What causes the face inversion effect? *Journal of Experimental Psychology: Human Perception and Performance, 21,* 628–634.

Farah, M. J., Wilson, Drain, H. M., & Tanaka, J. W. (1998). What is "special" about face perception? *Psychological Review, 105,* 482–498.

Galaburda, A., & Bellugi, U. (chap. 5). Cellular and molecular cortical neuroanatomy in Williams Syndrome.

Geisser, S., & Greenhouse, S. (1959). On methods in the analysis of profile data. *Psychometrika, 24,* 95–112.

Harter, R., Ainne, C. J., & Schroeder, C. (1984). Hemispheric differences in event-related potential measures of selective attention. Sixth international conference on event-related slow potentials of the brain (EPIC VI): Cognition, and information processing. *Annals of the New York Academy of Sciences, 425,* 210–211.

Haxby, J. V., Grady, C. L., Horwitz, B., Salerno, J., Ungerleider, L. G., Mishkin, M., & Schapiro, M. B. (1993). Dissociation of object and spatial visual processing pathways in human extrastriate cortex. In B. Gulyas, D. Ottoson, & P. E. Roland (Eds.), *Functional organization of the human visual cortex* (pp. 329–340). Oxford: Pergamon Press.

Haxby, J., Grady, C. L., Horwitz, B., Ungerleider, L. G., Mishkin, M., Carson, R. E., Herscovitch, P., Schapiro, M. B., & Rappoport, S. I. (1991). Dissociation of object and spatial visual processing pathways in human extratriate cortex. *Proceedings of the National Academy of Sciences U.S.A., 88,* 1621–1625.

Haxby, J. V., Horwitz, B., Ungerleider, L. G., Maisog, J. M., Pietrini, P., & Grady, C. L. (1994). The functional organization of human extrastriate cortex: A PET-rCBF study of selective attention to faces and locations. *Journal of Neuroscience, 14,* 6336–6353.

Hécaen, H., Goldblum, M. C., Masure, M. C., & Ramier, A. M. (1974). A new observation of object agnosia: Is the specific deficit for the visual modality one of association or of categorization? *Neuropsychologia, 12,* 447–464.

Hillyard, S., & Kutas, M. (1983). Electrophysiology of cognitive processing. *Annual Review of Psychology, 34,* 33–61.

Hillyard, S., Mangun, G., Woldorff, M., & Luck, S. (1995). Neural systems mediating selective attention. In M. Gazzaniga (Ed.), *The cognitive neurosciences* (pp. 665–682). Cambridge, MA: MIT Press.

Jernigan, T. L., & Bellugi, U. (1994). Neuroanatomical distinctions between Williams and Down syndromes. In S. Broman & J. Grafman (Eds.), *Atypical cognitive deficits in developmental disorders: Implications in brain function* (pp. 57–66). Hillsdale, NJ: Erlbaum.

Jones, W., Hickok, G., & Lai, Z. (1998). Does face processing rely on intact visual-spatial abilities? Evidence from Williams syndrome. *Cognitive Neuroscience Society Abstract Program, 80,* 67.

Jones, W., Rossen, M. L., Hickok, G., Jernigan, T., & Bellugi, U. (1995). Links between behavior and brain: Brain morphological correlates of language, face, and auditory processing in Williams syndrome. *Society for Neuroscience Abstracts, 21,* 1926.

Kanwisher, N., McDermott, J., & Chun, M. M. (1997). The fusiform area: A module in human extrastriate cortex specialized for face perception. *Journal of Neuroscience, 17,* 4302–4311.

Kanwisher, N., Tong, F., & Nakayama, K. (1998). The effect of face inversion on the human fusiform face area. *Cognition, 68,* B1–B11.

Kutas, M., & Hillyard, S. (1980). Event-related potentials to semantically inappropriate and surprisingly large words. *Biological Psychology, 11,* 99–116.

Leehy, S., Carey, S., Diamond, R., & Cahn, A. (1978). Upright and inverted faces: The right hemisphere knows the difference. *Cortex, 14,* 411–419.

Levy, J., Trevarthen, C., & Sperry, R. W. (1972). Perception of bilateral chimeric figures following hemispheric deconnexion. *Brain, 95,* 61–78.

Magnussen, S., Sunde, B., & Dyrnes, S. (1994). Patterns of perceptual asymmetry in processing facial expression. *Cortex, 30,* 215–229.

Mangun, G. R., & Hillyard, S. A. (1991). Modulations of sensory-evoked brain potentials provide evidence for changes in perceptual processing during visual-spatial priming. *Journal of Experimental Psychology: Human Perception, 17,* 1057–1074.

Mangun, G. R., Hillyard, S. A., & Luck, S. J. (1993). Electrocortical substrates of visual selective attention. In D. Meyer & S. Kornblum (Eds.), *Attention and Performance, 14,* 219–243.

McCarthy, G., Puce, A., Belger, A., & Allison, T. (1999). Electrophysiological studies of human face perception: II. Response properties of face-specific potentials generated in occipitotemporal cortex. *Cerebral Cortex, 9,* 431–444.

McCarthy, G., Puce, A., Gore, J. C., & Allison, T. (1997). Face-specific processing in the human fusiform gyrus. *Journal of Cognitive Neuroscience, 9,* 605–610.

McCarthy, G., & Wood, C. C. (1985). Scalp distributions of event-related potentials: An ambiguity associated with analysis of variance models. *Electroencephalography and Clinical Neurophysiology, 59,* 203–208.

Mills, D. L. (1998). Electrophysiological markers of Williams syndrome. In U. Bellugi (Ed.), Bridging cognition, brain and genes: Evidence from genetically based syndromes. *Cognitive Neuroscience Society 1998 Annual Meeting Abstract Program,* 10.

Mooney, C. M. (1957). Age in the development of closure ability in children. *Canadian Journal of Psychology, 11,* 216–226.

Moscovitch, M., Winocur, G., & Behrmann, M. (1997). What is special about face recognition? Nineteen experiments on a person with visual object agnosia and dyslexia but normal face recognition. *Journal of Cognitive Neuroscience, 9,* 555–604.

Neville, H. J., Coffey, S. A., Holcomb, P. J., & Tallal, P. (1993). The neurobiology of sensory and language processing in language-impaired children. *Journal of Cognitive Neuroscience, 5,* 235–253.

Neville, H. J., Mills, D. L., & Bellugi, U. (1994). Effects of altered auditory sensitivity and age of language acquisition on the development of language-relevant neural systems: Preliminary studies of Williams syndrome. In S. Broman & J. Grafman (Eds.), *Atypical cognitive deficits in developmental disorders: Implications for brain function* (pp. 67–83). Hillsdale, NJ: Erlbaum.

Polich, J., Ellerson, P. C., & Cohen, J. (1996). P300 stimulus intensity, modality, and probability. *International Journal of Psychophysiology, 23,* 55–62.

Puce, A., Allison, T., Gore, J. C., & McCarthy, G. (1995). Face-sensitive regions in human extrastriate cortex studied by functional MRI. *Journal of Neurophysiology, 74,* 1192–1199.

Puce, A., Allison, T., & McCarthy, G. (1999). Electrophysiological studies of human face perception: III. Effects of top-down processing on face-specific potentials. *Cerebral Cortex, 9,* 445–458.

Reiss, A., Eliez, S., Schmitt, E., Strouss, E., Lai, Z., Jones, W., & Bellugi, U. (chap. 4). Neuroanatomy of Williams Syndrome: A high-resolution MRI study.

Rhodes, G. (1985). Lateralized processes in face recognition. *British Journal of Psychology, 76,* 249–271.

Rossen, M. L., Jones, W., Wang, P. P., & Klima, E. S. (1995). Face processing: Remarkable sparing in Williams syndrome. Special Issue, *Genetic Counseling, 6,* 138–140.

Schweinberger, S. R., & Sommer, W. (1991). Contributions of stimulus encoding and memory search to right hemisphere superiority in face recognition: Behavioral and electrophysiological evidence. *Neuropsychologia, 29,* 389–413.

Schweinberger, S. R., Sommer, W., & Stiller, R. M. (1994). Event-related potentials and models of performance asymmetries in face and word recognition. *Neuropsychologia, 32,* 175–191.

Sergent, J. (1986). Methodological constraints on neuropsychological studies of face perception in normals. In R. Bruyer (Ed.), *The neuropsychology of face perception and facial expression* (pp. 91–124). Hillsdale, NJ: Erlbaum.

Sergent, J., Ohta, S., & MacDonald, B. (1992). Functional neuroanatomy of face and object processing. A positron emission tomography study. *Brain, 115,* 15–36.

Tanaka, J. W., & Farah, M. (1991). Second-order relational properties and the inversion effect: Testing a theory of face perception. *Perception and Psychophysics, 50,* 367–372.

Tukey, J. W. (1997). *Exploratory data analysis.* Reading, MA: Addison-Wesley.

Valentine, T. (1988). Upside-down faces: A review of the effect of inversion upon face recognition. *British Journal of Psychology, 79,* 471–491.

Warrington, E. K. (1984). *Warrington recognition memory test.* Windsor, England: Nfer-Nelson Publishing.

Wechsler, D. (1974). *Wechsler intelligence scale for children—revised.* San Antonio, TX: The Psychological Corporation.

Wechsler, D. (1981). *Wechsler adult intelligences scale—revised.* San Antonio, TX: The Psychological Corporation.

Wojciulik, E., Kanwisher, N., & Driver, J. (1998). Covert visual attention modulates face-specific activity in the human fusiform gyrus. *Journal of Neurophysiology, 79,* 1574–1578.

Yin, R. K. (1969). Looking at upside-down faces. *Journal of Experimental Psychology, 81,* 141–145.

Yin, R. K. (1970). Face recognition by brain-injured patients: A dissociable ability? *Neuropsychologia, 8,* 395–402.

4 Neuroanatomy of Williams Syndrome: A High-Resolution MRI Study

Allan L. Reiss, Stephan Eliez, J. Eric Schmitt, Erica Straus, Zona Lai, Wendy Jones, and Ursula Bellugi

Williams syndrome (WMS), a genetic condition resulting from a contiguous deletion on the long arm of chromosome 7, is associated with a relatively consistent profile of neurocognitive and neurobehavioral features. The distinctiveness and regularity of the profile of learning and behavioral characteristics in this genetic condition suggests that underlying neurobiological correlates may be identifiable. In this chapter, we report initial findings derived from a high-resolution neuroimaging study of 14 young adult subjects with WMS and an individually matched normal control group. Compared to controls, subjects with WMS were noted to have decreased overall brain and cerebral volumes, relative preservation of cerebellar and superior temporal gyrus (STG) volumes, and disproportionate volume reduction of the brainstem. Analyses also suggested that the pattern of cerebral lobe proportions in WMS may be altered compared to normal controls with a greater ratio of frontal to posterior (parietal+occipital) tissue. Assessment of tissue composition indicated that, relative to controls, individuals with WMS have relative preservation of cerebral gray matter volume and disproportionate reduction in cerebral white matter volume. However, within the cerebral gray matter tissue compartment, the right occipital lobe was noted to have excess volume loss. Combined with our growing knowledge of the function of genes in the commonly deleted region for WMS, more detailed information regarding the structure and function of the WMS brain will provide a unique opportunity for elucidating meaningful correlations amongst genetic, neurobiological, and neurobehavioral factors in humans.

Introduction

The study of discrete genetic causes of cognitive and behavioral dysfunction in humans presents a unique opportunity to expand our knowledge of associations among specific genetic factors, brain development and function, and neurobehavioral outcome. Of the many genetic conditions that provide a model for furthering our knowledge in this regard, few are as intriguing or enigmatic as Williams syndrome (WMS). This condition, originally named to represent a syndromic constellation of developmental, physical, cognitive, and behavioral features, is now known to be caused by a contiguous deletion on the long arm of chromosome 7 (band 7q11.23) (Ewart et al., 1993; Korenberg et al., 1996; Korenberg, Chen, Lai, et al., 1997a; Korenberg, Chen, Mirchell, & Sun, 1997b; Korenberg et al., this volume; Lowery et al., 1995).

Despite the presence of a number of physical features and medical problems that are of potential clinical significance in persons with WMS, such as failure to thrive, infantile hypercalcemia, and cardiac or vascular malformations (Morris, Demsey, Leonard, Dilts, & Blackburn, 1988), sequelae of central nervous system dysfunction predominate as the most impeding in an affected individual's daily functioning. In particular, individuals with WMS usually function within the mild to moderate mentally retarded range of intelligence. However, cognitive function is typically uneven with the characteristic profile including relative strengths in particular components of expressive language, musical abilities and face processing, and relative weakness in nonverbal functions such as spatial cognition and visual-motor abilities (Bellugi, Bihrle, Jernigan, Trauner, & Doherty, 1990; Bellugi, Wang, & Jernigan, 1993; Bellugi, Lichtenberger, Mills, Galaburda, & Korenberg, 1999a; Bellugi, Mills, Jernigan, Hickok, & Galaburda, 1999b; Bellugi et al., chap. 1; Hickok, Bellugi, & Jones, 1995a; Lenhoff, Wang, Greenberg, & Bellugi, 1997).

The presence of a predictable neurobehavioral phenotype, coupled with the availability of increasingly sophisticated technology for assessing brain structure and function, led to preliminary brain imaging studies in individuals with WMS. Although these studies often employed comparison subjects with another specific genetic condition, Down syndrome, as well as normal controls, the current discussion focuses on the latter comparison, as it is most applicable to the data provided in the present study. Initial findings from these preliminary imaging studies suggested that the brains of individuals with WMS were reduced in volume overall compared to normal controls (Jernigan & Bellugi, 1990; Jernigan, Bellugi, Sowell, Doherty, & Hesselink, 1993). However, brain volume reductions in WMS, like cognitive abilities, appeared uneven on a regional basis with relative preservation of temporal-limbic and cerebellar volumes (Jernigan et al., 1993), and superior temporal auditory cortex (Hickok et al., 1995b). A recent preliminary report also suggested that gray matter might be preferentially preserved in WMS (Harris-Collazo, Archibald, Lai, Bellugi, & Jernigan, 1997).

However, previous imaging studies investigating brain structure in WMS have limitations. First, these studies typically employed small group sizes. Second, much of the volumetric-anatomical data on subjects with WMS and controls were established with image acquisitions characterized by relatively low resolution (e.g., 5-mm brain slices with 2.5-mm gaps in-between slices) (Jernigan & Bellugi, 1990; Jernigan et al., 1993) as compared to current imaging techniques that permit 1–2-mm resolution on a routine basis. Third, previous studies emphasized comparisons between WMS and Down syndrome. This made it difficult to determine whether group differences should be attributed to abnormal brain morphology in the WMS group, the Down syndrome group, or both. Accordingly, the need for further studies to investigate brain structure and function in this important genetic condition is great, and promises to reveal information of significance to a broader understanding of gene-brain-behavior associations in humans.

The data presented here represents our laboratory's initial collaborative work on elucidating the neuroanatomical basis of the cognitive and behavioral features associated with WMS. Data from previous imaging and postmortem studies reporting on small numbers of subjects with WMS, provided a focal point from which initial questions and hypotheses could be generated. Specifically, in this initial imaging study of WMS, we sought preliminary answers to the following questions:

1. Is decreased brain volume a consistent feature of WMS?

2. Is there relative sparing of the frontal lobe and cerebellum, and disproportionate reduction of parietal and occipital regions, during brain development in WMS?

3. Is white matter disproportionately affected and gray matter preferentially preserved during brain development in WMS?

4. Are relative strengths in specific language and music abilities in subjects with WMS reflected in preserved development of the superior temporal gyrus (STG), a region known to be of importance to both of these cognitive domains?

In this study, we report on preliminary information derived from a comparison of 14 young adult subjects with WMS to a normal control group individually matched for gender and age.

Results

Overall Brain and Tissue Volumes in WMS

As shown in the Table 4.1 and Figure 4.1, total brain volume was decreased 13%, on average, in subjects with WMS compared to controls ($F = 14.4$, $p < .001$). However, this reduction in volume did not extend across the brain in a proportional manner. Specifically, while cerebral volume showed a 13% decrease in subjects with WMS ($F = 14.9$, $p < .001$), cerebellar volume was decreased to a lesser extent (7%). Moreover, the cerebellar volume difference between the two groups was not significant ($F = 3.7$, $p < .10$). When a variable reflecting the ratio of cerebellar volume to cerebral volume was created, WMS subjects were noted to have significantly higher ratios compared to controls ($z = 2.4$, $p < .02$) (Figure 4.2). In contrast to the cerebellar findings, brainstem tissue volumes were significantly reduced (20%) in individuals with WMS compared to controls ($F = 27.5$; $p < .0001$). This reduction in brainstem tissue volume was proportionally

Table 4.1
Global and Regional Brain Volumes in WMS and Normal Controls

	WMS (n = 14)		Controls (n = 14)		WMS/
	mean	SD	mean	SD	Control (%)
Age	28.7	8.9	29.0	9.0	
Total Brain Volume	1183.7	100.1	1356.7	138.2	87.2
Total Gray Matter	629.0	54.0	677.3	90.0	92.9
Total White Matter	410.6	57.1	520.7	68.3	78.9
Total CSF	144.1	36.4	158.7	21.9	90.8
Total Cerebral Volume	1025.1	90.0	1181.3	121.5	86.8
Cerebrum gray	535.6	46.7	577.0	74.3	92.8
Sub-cortical gray	38.4	4.3	40.5	4.9	94.8
Cerebrum White	364.0	51.6	466.8	62.2	78.0
Cerebrum CSF	125.5	31.7	137.5	19.7	91.3
Lateral Ventricle CSF	10.1	3.6	12.6	4.0	80.2
Frontal lobe tissue	330.3	34.4	375.6	43.6	87.9
Frontal lobe gray	193.1	19.3	205.5	27.3	94.0
Frontal lobe white	137.2	20.3	170.1	23.3	80.7
Parietal lobe tissue	225.1	23.7	257.7	31.8	87.3
Parietal lobe gray	127.6	12.9	133.3	18.5	95.7
Parietal lobe white	97.5	14.1	124.4	19.5	78.4
Temporal lobe tissue	170.6	12.2	200.2	23.0	85.2
Temporal lobe gray	116.1	8.6	125.8	15.4	92.3
Temporal lobe white	54.5	7.9	74.4	11.6	73.3
Occipital lobe tissue	97.5	13.2	124.3	19.5	78.4
Occipital lobe gray	60.3	8.0	72.0	12.7	83.8
Occipital lobe white	37.2	7.3	52.3	10.1	71.1
Total Cerebellar Volume	134.2	11.6	144.5	16.6	92.9
Cerebellum tissue	118.6	9.7	127.5	15.0	93.0
Cerebellar Gray	84.2	8.3	88.3	15.4	95.4
Cerebellar White	34.5	6.6	39.2	7.9	88.0
Cerebellar CSF	15.6	5.2	17.0	2.8	91.8
Total Brainstem Volume	24.5	3.1	30.8	2.8	79.5
Brainstem tissue	21.4	2.7	26.6	2.6	80.5
Brainstem CSF	3.1	0.7	4.2	0.8	73.8
Sup. Temp. Gyrus (STG)					
STG Tissue	31.8	2.7	33.4	3.0	95.2
STG Gray	22.6	1.7	22.0	2.4	102.7
STG White	9.2	1.6	11.4	1.6	80.7

Note: All volumes are in cubic centimeters (cm³)
The table shows comparative brain volumes in 14 subjects with WMS as compared to a group of age- and gender-matched normal controls. The last column shows the ratio (proviced as a percentage) of the average WMS volume to the average control subject volume. Nonproportional differences between the two groups are illustrated by the 12 percent reduction in frontal-lobe tissue volume as compared to a nearly 22 percent reduction for occipital-lobe tissue volume in subjects with WMS. Cerebellar volume is reduced only 7 percent in subjects with WMS relative to normal controls.

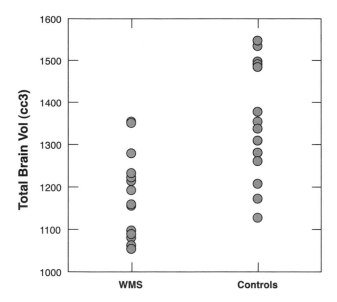

Brain Volume in Williams Syndrome and Normal Controls

Figure 4.1
Average brain volumes in subjects with WMS were decreased 13 percent compared to controls. All values are in cubic centimeters (cm³).

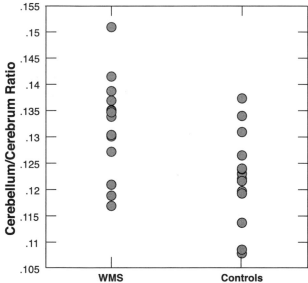

Ratio of Cerebellum to Cerebrum Volume

Figure 4.2
The greater ratio observed in subjects with WMS compared to control subjects represents a relative preservation of cerebellar volume in comparison to cerebral volume.

greater ($F = 8.8$, $p < .007$) than that observed for reduction in overall brain tissue volume in the WMS group.

Analysis of cerebral tissue components revealed significant differences in relative gray and white matter tissue composition between the groups. Using total cerebral volume and age as covariates in an analysis of covariance (ANCOVA), subjects with WMS were shown to have relative "sparing" of their cerebral gray matter volume compared to controls ($F = 5.3$, $p = .03$), and disproportionate reduction in cerebral white matter volume ($F = 4.3$, $p = .05$). CSF volume was reduced in a manner proportional to overall cerebral volume in the WMS group. Using a similar ANCOVA with total cerebellar volume and age as covariates, the pattern of gray matter sparing or disproportionate white matter reduction was not observed in the cerebellum of individuals with WMS. Similarly, neither subcortical gray matter volume nor lateral ventricular volume was observed to be reduced or increased in a disproportionate manner compared to the respective overall cerebral tissue volume.

Brain Asymmetry in WMS

Repeated measures analysis of variance (ANOVA) revealed a significant group by side difference for occipital-lobe tissue ($F = 5.0$, $p < .04$ for the group × side interaction term). Specifically, as opposed to control subjects who showed relative symmetry in occipital-lobe tissue volumes for the right and left sides (62.5 and 61.8 cm³, respectively), the WMS group showed leftward predominance for this region (47.3 and 50.2 cm³, respectively). This finding appeared to be secondary to a left > right shift in gray matter of the occipital lobe in the WMS group ($F = 4.6$, $p < .05$) as opposed to white matter ($F = 2.5$, $p = .13$). No other variable assessed suggested group differences in asymmetry including hemispheric and individual lobe gray and white matter volumes, subcortical gray volumes, and ventricular volumes. These findings indicate that the brains of individuals with WMS show abnormal patterns of asymmetry in the occipital lobe, primarily due to an abnormal leftward predominance of gray matter.

Cerebral Lobe Proportions in WMS

Multivariate analysis of covariance (MANCOVA) was initially utilized to determine whether individuals with WMS demonstrate an atypical *pattern* of cerebral morphology. This analysis used group as the main effect (i.e., WMS vs. Controls), total cerebral tissue as a covariate, and the combined right and left tissue volumes of each the four lobes of the brain as the dependent variables (i.e., frontal-lobe tissue, parietal-lobe tissue, temporal-lobe tissue, and occipital-lobe tissue). The F-value for the main effect of group was not significant (Wilks' lambda $F = 0.92$, $p < 0.50$) indicating that individuals with WMS did not possess a unique pattern of cerebral tissue morphology in comparison to the control group. However, to further explore this issue, a variable was constructed that consisted of the ratio of frontal-lobe tissue volume to the combined tissue volumes of the parietal and occipital lobes. Nonparametric analysis using this variable indicated that the WMS group showed larger ratios compared to controls ($z = 2.2$, $p < .03$) suggesting that cerebral lobe brain proportions may be aberrant in WMS.

Given the disproportionate effect of WMS on gray and white matter volumes, MANCOVAs were also utilized to investigate patterns of tissue-specific brain development. For example, analysis of gray matter morphology used total cerebral gray matter and age as covariates, and the combined right and left gray matter volumes of each the four lobes of the brain as dependent variables. The white matter analysis was identical with the exception of using white matter volumes as the covariate and dependent variables. A statistical trend was observed for the gray matter lobe MANCOVA (Wilks' lambda $F = 2.27$, $p < .10$), thus suggesting that the pattern of gray matter cerebral morphology in WMS was distinct from that observed in controls; the MANCOVA for cerebral white matter was not significant (Wilks' lambda $F = 0.73$, $p < 0.60$).

Further exploratory analyses were conducted for possible group differences in gray matter lobe volumes because of the statistical trend observed in the gray matter MANCOVA and because differences in patterns of asymmetry for occipital-lobe gray matter were previously noted between subjects with WMS and controls. Specifically, these analyses included (1) evaluation of individual ANCOVA components comprising the gray matter lobe MANCOVA described in the preceding paragraph, and (2) assessment of individual right- and left-occipital-lobe gray matter volumes using total cerebral gray matter and age as covariates. These analyses indicated that parietal-lobe gray matter volume tended to be disproportionately increased in subjects with WMS ($F = 5.6$, $p < .03$) while occipital-lobe gray matter volume was disproportionately reduced ($F = 4.9$, $p < .04$) compared to controls. Analysis of separate right and left occipital gray matter volumes indicated that disproportionate volume loss in this region was predominately on the right side ($F = 10.4$, $p < .004$) as opposed to the left ($F = 1.8$, $p < .20$).

Superior Temporal Gyrus

ANCOVA was used to assess the relative volume of the STG, and its gray and white matter components. These analyses used group as the main effect, age and total cerebral tissue, gray or white matter volume respectively, as covariates, and STG tissue volumes (total tissue, gray matter, and white matter, respectively) as dependent variables. The analyses revealed that, after statistically adjusting for overall cerebral gray matter volume, gray matter STG volumes in subjects with WMS were proportionally *larger* compared to controls ($F = 4.7$, $p = .05$). In fact, the unadjusted mean gray matter volume ($\pm$ *SD*) for the WMS group ($22.6 \pm 1.7 \, cm^3$) was slightly larger than that observed

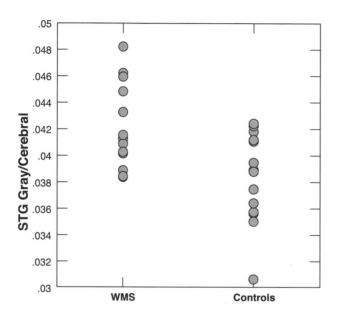

Figure 4.3
The greater ratio observed in subjects with WMS compared to control subjects represents a relative preservation of gray matter volume of the superior temporal gyrus in comparison to overall cerebral gray matter volume.

for the normal control group (22.0 ± 2.4 cm³). This between-group difference is reflected in Figure 4.3, that shows the STG gray/cerebral gray ratios in the two groups.

Age-Associated Effects

ANOVA was utilized to investigate potential group differences in brain morphology associated with age. In these analyses, a group by age interaction term was the primary effect of interest. Dependent variables of interest included cerebral and cerebellar total tissue, gray, white, and CSF volumes, and lateral ventricular CSF and subcortical gray matter volumes. The interaction term was significant only for ventricular CSF volume ($F = 12.8$, $p = .002$). Specifically, analysis of age-related changes by group showed that the trajectory of CSF volume in WMS was increasing with age ($r = 0.68$, $p < .008$) compared to a nonsignificant trend for ventricular CSF volume to decrease with age in the control group ($r = -0.51$, $p < .10$). A statistical trend also was observed for total cerebral CSF volume ($F = 4.1$, $p = .06$). Individual group-age-by-volume analysis showed a pattern similar to that observed for ventricular CSF volume. The WMS group demonstrated increasing cerebral CSF volume with age ($r = 0.61$, $p < .02$), while the control group showed no apparent correlation between these variables ($r = .05$, $p = 0.85$).

Discussion

It is clear that precise characterization of anomalous brain development in WMS will eventually require longitudinal comparison of large numbers of young individuals with this condition to persons with both nonspecific as well as other specific causes of developmental disability, in addition to typically developing age-, and developmental-age matched controls. Nevertheless, the findings presented here provide preliminary direction for future studies.

In this study, subjects with WMS were found to have smaller brain volumes than controls, with relative preservation of cerebellar volume (see Figure 4.4). An additional finding was the occurrence of disproportionate reduction in brainstem tissue volume in

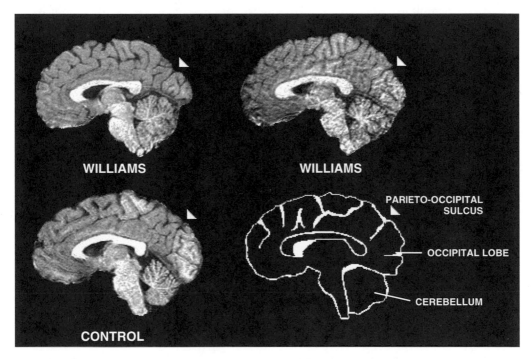

Figure 4.4
Occipital-lobe reduction in WMS and relative preservation of cerebellar size. Comparable sagittal MRI brain images from two subjects with WMS and a normal control. The images demonstrate that the occipital lobe, separated from the parietal lobe by the parietal-occipital sulcus (see triangle), is greatly reduced in the subjects with WMS. Relative preservation of cerebellar size in WMS relative to controls also is shown.

subjects with WMS. The results pertaining to cerebral and cerebellar volumes replicate findings from a previous study that assessed brain morphology in nine subjects with WMS (one subject overlapping with the present study), compared to six subjects with Down syndrome and 21 normal controls (Jernigan et al., 1993).

The presence of unusual patterns of brain morphology in the posterior fossa of individuals with WMS is of potential significance to recent reports describing genes present in the commonly deleted region on chromosome 7q. In particular, FZD3, a human homologue of the *Drosophila* gene "frizzled," is thought to be involved in early development of the mammalian central nervous system, particularly the midbrain, pons and cerebellum (Wang et al., 1997). This apparent convergence of findings from imaging and molecular genetic studies of WMS suggests that future research should focus on the association of FZD3 and this brain region as a potential contributor to the neurobehavioral phenotype occurring in individuals with WMS.

Qualitative postmortem examination of gross neuroanatomy from persons with WMS has suggested that a pattern of frontal sparing and disproportionate posterior (parietal-occipital) reductions in cerebral volume may characterize the condition (see Figure 4.4) (Bellugi et al., 1999b; Galaburda & Bellugi, chap. 5; Galaburda, Wang, Bellugi, & Rosen, 1994). The initial statistical analyses used in the present study provided only partial quantitative support for this hypothesis. While the MANCOVA for cerebral-lobe tissue failed to demonstrate a morphological pattern that differentiated subjects with WMS from controls, a variable representing the ratio of frontal-lobe volume to parietal + occipital-lobe volumes suggested the possibility of abnormal cerebral proportions in WMS. Further, occipital-lobe gray matter volume, particularly on the right, was noted to be decreased in the WMS group compared to controls while parietal-lobe gray matter volume was noted to be increased. These results are generally consistent with earlier imaging studies reporting reductions in brain volumes across cerebral regions in subjects with WMS (Jernigan et al., 1993); these subjects also were described as having relative "sparing" of frontal regions when compared to subjects with Down syndrome.

Relative preservation of gray matter and disproportionate reduction in white matter in subjects with WMS compared to normal controls is a particularly intriguing finding of the present study. This finding could result from alteration of any of a number of progressive or regressive events occurring during normal central nervous system development. These include cellular proliferation, migration and programmed death, growth and refinement of the neuropil, and myelination. A previous study, examining gray-white proportions in subjects with WMS, failed to detect differences from normal subjects (Jernigan et al., 1993). However, scan acquisition parameters for this prior study differed significantly from those utilized in the present study. In particular, image slice thickness in the earlier study was five times larger than the 1.5-mm slices utilized here. Increased slice thickness (and accordingly, voxel size) is associated with greater volume averaging artifacts occurring in image voxels that contain nonhomogenous tissues, thus potentially resulting in loss of image resolution and accuracy of tissue segmentation. The hypothesis that increased slice thickness, and thus, greater volume averaging, may explain the discrepancy in findings of this earlier study is supported by a more recent report from this same group. Specifically, using higher resolution scans that decreased artifact resulting from volume averaging, Harris-Collazo et al. (1997) reported that gray matter proportions appeared increased in a group of seven young adult subjects with WMS when plotted on a scattergram showing the proportion of gray matter as a function of age in normal controls.

If confirmed as a consistent feature of this genetic condition, the finding of abnormal proportions of gray and white matter may also help guide the investigation of the function of other proteins resulting from genes deleted in persons with WMS. For example, the protein kinase resulting from the gene LIMK1, located in the commonly deleted WMS region, has been hypothesized to play a role in intracellular signaling, and synapse formation and maintenance in the central nervous system (Wang, Frenzel, Wen, & Falls, 1998). Similarly, syntaxin, the protein product of another gene deleted in WMS (STX1A), is thought to be involved in exocytosis of neurotransmitters from neurons (Nakayama et al., 1998). More detailed information regarding the role of these and other genes in the WMS critical region in human brain structure and function will provide a unique opportunity for elucidating meaningful correlations amongst genetic, neurobiological, and neurobehavioral factors in this genetic condition.

One brain area found to be preserved in size in subjects with WMS in this study, as well as in past imaging investigations of this condition (Hickok et al., 1995a; Hickok et al., 1995b), is the superior temporal region. This region of the brain is thought to be important in the perception and processing of music (Liegeois-Chauvel, Peretz, Babai, Laguitton, & Chauvel, 1998; Zatorre, Evans, & Meyer, 1994), as well as its well-known function in auditory and language processing (Demonet et al., 1992; Price et al., 1992; Schlosser et al., 1998). It is of potential interest that the gray matter volume of this region appears most preserved in individuals with WMS, given their relative cognitive strengths in both of these domains of cognitive processing and function. However, it would be premature to directly relate relatively larger gray matter volume of the superior temporal region in WMS to the cognitive profile exhibited by persons with this condition. As opposed to "endowing" persons with WMS with language and musical abilities, larger superior temporal gray matter volume in WMS might, alternatively, be secondary to consistently greater use of these cognitive skills over time resulting in larger cortical representation (Pantev et al., 1998) and corresponding increased neuropil (Sirevaag, Black, Shafron, & Greenough, 1988). Longitudinal structural and functional imaging studies of young children with WMS are likely to help resolve this question.

Finally, in contrast to controls, age-related increases in total cerebral and, more specifically, lateral ventricular CSF, were noted in subjects with WMS. Positive correlations between CSF volume and age in subjects with WMS were not accompanied by significant negative correlations between age and tissue in this study. However, as CSF volume is significantly smaller than either gray or white matter volumes, relatively small, nonsignificant reduction in tissue volume over time could theoretically result in a proportionally larger, complementary change in CSF volume that is statistically significant. Longitudinal imaging studies of a large cohort of subjects with WMS will be essential in helping to resolve the question of whether abnormal age associated changes in neuroanatomy exist in WMS. If confirmed, clinical correlates of these age-related changes will be of great importance. For example, while WMS is clearly not a typical neurodegenerative disorder, recent studies suggest that some behavioral problems may intensify as some affected individuals enter adulthood (Gosch & Pankau, 1997).

Recent Findings

Continuing analyses of structural neuroimaging data are suggesting that, compared to normal controls, individuals with WMS have a unique profile of neuroanatomical variation with a predisposition for particular volume and shape abnormalities. Recent findings have implicated a reduced volume of posterior cerebral regions, with an abnormal cerebral shape, shown by a quantitative "bending angle" analyses, a measure of the curvature of an object in two dimensions. Data from 20 individuals with WMS and 20 age-matched controls were analyzed. The results indicate that individuals with WMS have significantly larger bending angles for both the left and the right cerebral hemispheres. These differences are similar to those described in Galaburda and Bellugi (chap. 5, this volume) and are likely due to decreased volume of the parietal occipital regions. Since parietal and occipital lobes are implicated in visuospatial processing, this is congruent with the poor visuospatial abilities observed in individuals with WMS (Schmitt, Eliez, Bellugi, & Reiss, 2001).

It is likely that the neuromorphologic variations observed in WMS, a syndrome with a proven genetic origin, are caused by aberrant brain development. Paralleling the cerebral findings, the bending angle of the corpus callosum was significantly larger in the WMS group. As with the cerebral findings, the observed differences may be due to a reduction in the posterior cortical regions. In quantitative analyses of the corpus callosum area, the posterior regions of the corpus callosum (isthmus and splenium) were significantly reduced in WMS relative to the control group. Interestingly, the isthmus and the splenium contain the vast majority of white matter tracts that bilaterally connect the visual and visual association areas of the brain. The anterior three-fifths of the corpus callosum, which connect the frontal and temporal lobes, were relatively preserved. The overall shape of the corpus callosum in WMS follows the general morphological trends previously observed in this condition: relatively preserved anterior regions with decreases in size posteriorly. Both the corpus callosum and the cerebral hemispheres develop in a rostrocaudal direction. Premature termination of brain development along the rostrocaudal axis could produce cortical shapes much like that of the WMS subjects reported here. Therefore, the neuroanatomical findings reported here appear to concur with the well-known visuospatial difficulties ascribed to WMS and suggest a possible neuroanatomical correlate (Bellugi et al., chap. 1). This also agrees with the known neurobehavioral profile of WMS, in which relative preservations of frontal and temporal lobe functions such as language and affect are found (Schmitt, Eliez, Warsofsky, Bellugi, & Reiss, 2001).

One of the most intriguing findings in morphometric analyses of the WMS brain is the suggestion of preservation of cerebellar volume, particularly in the cerebellar vermis. The neocerebellum, including the posterior vermis, is developmentally, evolutionarily, and histologically distinct from other cerebellar regions. Through phylogenetic history, the neocerebellum has grown relatively larger in mammals and particularly in humans, suggesting that this region may be involved in novel or cognitively complex functions. In a neuroimaging study, 20 normal controls and 20 WMS, the cerebellar vermis was divided into lobules I-V, VI-VII, and VIII-X and quantitatively measured. A recent study found that the posterior vermis is preserved in subjects with WMS when compared to normal controls; this region is, in fact, proportionally larger in WMS after adjusting for a measure of overall brain volume. Given the emerging evidence of a role for the posterior cerebellum in social and emotional behavior, the significantly increased size of the posterior vermis could be related to the hypersociability and positive affective behavior frequently observed in individuals with WMS.

Conclusion

This report represents the first in a series of investigations of the structure and function of the brain in individuals with WMS. Planned future studies will focus on limbic, mesial temporal, and subcortical regions, subregions of the cerebellum that have been reported to be particularly spared from volume reduction in this disorder (Wang, Hesselink, Jernigan, Doherty, & Bellugi, 1992), and the integrity and morphology of major white matter tracts, particularly the corpus callosum. Shape-based analyses of the cerebral lobes and their relation to the posterior fossa also are underway to more fully elucidate possible patterns of altered brain morphological development in individuals with WMS. Eventual correlation of neurocognitive and structural imaging findings with results obtained from functional imaging studies will be particularly important in elucidating the topography of neuroanatomical function and dysfunction underlying cognition and behavior in individuals affected with this enigmatic genetic condition.

Methods

Subjects

Fourteen individuals with WMS, (nine men and five women; mean age: 28.7 ± 8.9, range 19 to 44 years), and 14 normal controls matched individually for gender and age (mean age: 29.0 ± 9.0 years; range 20 to 48 years) were studied. All subjects gave informed consent in writing prior to participation and were physically healthy.

Subjects with WMS were tested as part of a large program project examining the associations among behavior, neurophysiology, neuroanatomy, and molecular genetics (see chapters, this volume). All subjects with WMS were diagnosed clinically by a medical geneticist or other physician familiar with the characteristic features of WMS prior to inclusion into the current study (Jones, 1990; Morris et al., 1988). Subjects were excluded from the study if they had a history of concurrent medical conditions not typically associated with WMS, particularly those with confounding medical or neurological consequences. All clinical diagnoses were confirmed by trained researchers using the Williams Syndrome Diagnostic Scoresheet, a screening measure developed by the medical advisory board of the Williams Syndrome Association (1994). In addition, the diagnosis of WMS was genetically confirmed in all of the subjects using the fluorescent in situ hybridization (FISH) test for a deletion of one copy of the elastin gene on chromosome 7, as part of the molecular genetic studies (Korenberg et al., chap. 6).

Imaging

Magnetic resonance images of each subject's brain were acquired with a GE-Signa 1.5 T scanner (General Electric, Milwaukee, WI). Sagittal images were acquired with a 3-D volumetric radio frequency spoiled gradient echo (SPGR) using the following scan parameters: TR = 24, TE = 5, flip angle = 45, NEX = 2, matrix size = 256 × 192, field of view = 24, slice thickness = 1.2 mm, 124 slices. Twenty-six of the 28 scans were acquired at the University of California, San Diego (UCSD) Medical Center Magnetic Resonance Imaging Institute. Two control scans were acquired at Stanford University using an identical pulse sequence and scanner. The SPGR image data were imported into the program *BrainImage* (Reiss, 1999) for semiautomated image processing analysis and quantification. These procedures have been described and validated elsewhere (Kaplan et al., 1997; Kates et al., 1999; Reiss et al., 1998; Subramanium, Hennessey, Rubin, Beach, & Reiss, 1997). Data resulting from this semiautomated image-processing pipeline is in the form of left and right gray matter, white matter, and cerebrospinal (CSF) fluid volumes for each of the cerebral lobes, a subcortical region including the basal ganglia and thalamus, the cerebellum, brainstem, and the lateral ventricles. An exception to the semiautomated parcellation scheme typically utilized in our laboratory was employed due to the fact that subjects with WMS have been noted to have possible shape differences in the posterior-inferior part of their brain. Therefore, to increase accuracy of the brain parcellation component of our image-processing pipeline, manual delineation of the cerebellum and brainstem was utilized using modifications of a previously established protocol (Aylward & Reiss, 1991). After measuring and masking out posterior fossa tissue, the remainder of the brain tissue (i.e., cerebrum) was subdivided into the respective cerebral lobes and subcortical regions with a Talairach-based automated parcellation procedure as previously described (Andreasen et al., 1996; Kaplan et al., 1997).

Manual delineation of the STG was also used to supplement the semiautomated procedure. The STG was measured in the rostral-caudal direction from images in the coronal plane that were derived from the original image dataset. This coronal dataset was oriented parallel to the plane defined by the anterior and posterior commissures. The boundaries of the STG were defined laterally by the cortical surface and medially by a line connecting the deepest extension of the superior temporal sulcus (STS) to the furthest extent of the inferior ramus of the sylvian fissure. The most anterior slice of the STG measured coincided with the halfway point between the head of the putamen and the anterior commissure. This designation ensured the operational exclusion of medial-temporal gyral tissue, which merges with the STG at the temporal pole. The most posterior slice of the STG measured coincided with the first slice where the crus of the fornix was clearly identified laterally from the pulvinar. Interrater reliability for measurement of the volume of this region as measured by the intraclass correlation coefficient was 0.96.

Data Analyses

Data were first examined for normality to conform to the assumptions of the parametric statistics employed. Uni- and multi-variate analyses of variance and co-variance were performed to analyze group differences in overall and regional brain volumes. In general, because the processes of myelinization and remodeling of the neuropil progress well into young adulthood, age was used as a standard covariate in all analyses in which either gray or white matter volumes were determined. Investigation of brain asymmetry utilized repeated measures ANOVA, which took diagnostic category as a between-subject factor and side (left vs. right) as a within-subject factor. The interaction effect (group × side) was used to determine group differences in asymmetry. Nonparametric statistical tests (Mann-Whitney U test) were used in all cases in which a ratio variable was assessed for group differences (e.g., cerebellar:cerebral ratio). A two-sided p value of .05 was chosen as the significant threshold except for analyses in which there was an a priori hypothesis in which case a one-sided test was utilized.

Notes

The research presented in this manuscript was supported from the following NIH grants: K02 MH01142 (ALR), R01 HD31715 (ALR), and P01 HD33113 (UB).

Illustrations and quotes not to be used without written permission from the author. Copyright Dr. Allan L. Reiss. Stanford, CA.

References

Andreasen, N. C., Rajarethinam, R., Cizadlo, T., Arndt, S., Swayze II, V. W., Flashman, L. A., O'Leary, D. S., Ehrhardt, J. C., & Yuh, W. T. (1996). Automatic atlas-based volume estimation of human brain regions from MR images. *Journal of Computer Assisted Tomography, 20,* 98–106.

Aylward, E. H., & Reiss, A. (1991). Area and volume measurement of posterior fossa structures in MRI. *Journal of Psychiatric Research, 25,* 159–168.

Bellugi, U., Bihrle, A., Jernigan, T., Trauner, D., & Doherty, S. (1990). Neuropsychological, neurological, and neuroanatomical profile of Williams syndrome. *American Journal of Medical Genetics, Supplement, 6,* 115–125.

Bellugi, U., Lichtenberger, L., Jones, W., Lai, Z., & St. George, M. (chap. 1). The neurocognitive profile of Williams Syndrome: A complex pattern of strengths and weaknesses.

Bellugi, U., Lichtenberger, L., Mills, D., Galaburda, A., & Korenberg, J. (1999a). Bridging cognition, brain and molecular genetics: Evidence from Williams syndrome. *Trends Neurosciences, 22,* 197–207.

Bellugi, U., Mills, D., Jernigan, T., Hickok, G., & Galaburda, A. (1999b). Linking cognition, brain structure and brain function in Williams syndrome. In H. Tager-Flusberg (Ed.), *Neurodevelopmental disorders: Contributions to a new framework from the cognitive neurosciences* (pp. 111–136). Cambridge, MA: MIT Press.

Bellugi, U., Wang, P., & Jernigan, T. (1993). Williams syndrome: An unusual neuropsychological profile. In S. Broman & J. Grafman (Eds.), *Atypical cognitive deficits in developmental disorders: Implications for brain function* (pp. 23–56). Hillsdale, NJ: Erlbaum.

Demonet, J. F., Chollet, F., Ramsay, S., Cardebat, D., Nespoulous, J. L., Wise, R., Rascol, A., & Frackowiak, R. (1992). The anatomy of phonological and semantic processing in normal subjects. *Brain, 115,* 1753–1768.

Ewart, A. K., Morris, C. A., Atkinson, D., Jin, W., Sternes, K., Spallone, P., Stock, A., Leppert, M., & Keating, M. (1993). Hemizygosity at the elastin locus in a developmental disorder, Williams syndrome. *Nature Genetics, 5,* 11–16.

Galaburda, A., & Bellugi, U. (chap. 5). Cellular and molecular cortical neuroanatomy in Williams Syndrome.

Galaburda, A., Wang, P. P., Bellugi, U., & Rosen, M. (1994). Cytoarchitectonic findings in a genetically-based disorder: Williams syndrome. *NeuroReport, 5,* 758–787.

Gosch, A., & Pankau, R. (1997). Personality characteristics and behaviour problems in individuals of different ages with Williams syndrome. *Developmental Medicine and Child Neurology, 39,* 527–533.

Harris-Callazo, M., Archibald, S., Lai, Z., Bellugi, U., & Jernigan, T. (1997). Morphological differences on quantitative MRI in Williams syndrome. *Society for Neuroscience,* New Orleans, LA.

Hickok, G., Bellugi, U., & Jones, W. (1995a). Asymmetrical ability [letter; comment]. *Science, 270,* 219–220.

Hickok, G., Neville, H., Mills, D., Jones, W., Rossen, M., & Bellugi, U. (1995b). Electrophysiological and quantitative MR analysis of the cortical auditory system in Williams syndrome. *Cognitive Neuroscience Society Abstracts, 2,* 66.

Jernigan, T. L., & Bellugi, U. (1990). Anomalous brain morphology on magnetic resonance images in Williams syndrome and Down syndrome. *Archives of Neurology, 47,* 529–533.

Jernigan, T. L., Bellugi, U., Sowell, E., Doherty, S., & Hesselink, J. R. (1993). Cerebral morphologic distinctions between Williams and Down syndromes. *Archives of Neurology, 50,* 186–191.

Jones, K. L. (1990). Williams syndrome: An historical perspective of its evolution, natural history, and etiology. *American Journal of Medical Genetics, Supplement, 6,* 89–96.

Kaplan, D. M., Liu, A. M., Abrams, M. T., Warsofsky, I. S., Kates, W. R., White, C. D., Kaufmann, W. E., & Reiss, A. (1997). Application of an automated parcellation method to the analysis of pediatric brain volumes. *Psychiatry Research, 76,* 15–27.

Kates, W. R., Warsofsky, I. S., Patwardhan, A., Abrams, M. T., Liu, A., Kaufmann, W. E., Naidu, S., & Reiss, A. L. (1999). Automated Talairach-based parcellation and measurement of cerebral lobes in children. *Psychiatry Research, 91,* 11–30.

Korenberg, J., Chen, X.-N., Hirota, H., Lai, Z., Bellugi, U., Burian, D., Roe, B., & Matsuoka, R. (chap. 6). Genome structure and cognitive map of Williams Syndrome.

Korenberg, J., Chen, X.-N., Lai, Z., Yimlamai, D., Bisighini, R., & Bellugi, U. (1997a). Williams syndrome: The search for the genetic origins of cognition. *American Journal of Human Genetics, 61,* 103.

Korenberg, J., Chen, X.-N., Mirchell, S., & Sun, Z. (1997b). The genomic organization of Williams syndrome. *International Behavioral Neuroscience Society Abstracts, 6,* 59.

Korenberg, J., Chen, X.-N., Mirchell, S., Sun, Z.-G., Hubert, R., Vataru, E., & Bellugi, U. (1996). The genomic organization of Williams syndrome. *American Journal of Human Genetics (Supplement), 59,* A306.

Lenhoff, H. M., Wang, P. P., Greenberg, F., & Bellugi, U. (1997). Williams syndrome and the brain. *Scientific American, 277,* 68–73.

Liegeois-Chauvel, C., Peretz, I., Babai, M., Laguitton, V., & Chauvel, P. (1998). Contribution of different cortical areas in the temporal lobes to music processing [see comments]. *Brain, 121,* 1853–1867.

Lowery, M. C., Morris, C. A., Ewart, A., Brothman, L. J., Zhu, X. L., Leonard, C., Carey, J., Keating, M., & Rothman, A. (1995). Strong correlation of elastin deletions, detected by FISH, with Williams syndrome: Evaluation of 235 patients. *American Journal of Human Genetics, 57,* 49–53.

Morris, C. A., Demsey, S. A., Leonard, C. O., Dilts, C., & Blackburn, B. L. (1988). Natural history of Williams syndrome: Physical characteristics. *Journal of Pediatrics, 113,* 318–326.

Nakayama, T., Matsuoka, R., Kimura, M., Hirota, H., Mikoshiba, K., Shimizu, Y., Shimizu, N., & Akagawa, K. (1998). Hemizygous deletion of the HPC-1/syntaxin 1A gene (STX1A) in patients with Williams syndrome. *Cytogenetics and Cell Genetics, 82,* 49–51.

Pantev, C., Oostenveld, R., Engelien, A., Ross, B., Roberts, L. E., & Hoke, M. (1998). Increased auditory cortical representation in musicians [see comments]. *Nature, 392,* 811–814.

Price, C., Wise, R., Ramsay, S., Friston, K., Howard, D., Patterson, K., & Frackowiak, R. (1992). Regional response differences within the human auditory cortex when listening to words. *Neuroscience Letters, 146,* 179–182.

Reiss, A. L. (1999). *BrainImage.* Stanford, CA: Stanford University.

Reiss, A. L., Hennessey, J. G., Rubin, M., Beach, L., Abrams, M. T., Warsofsky, I. S., Liu, A. M. C., et al. (1998). Reliability and validity of an algorithm for fuzzy tissue segmentation of magnetic resonance images. *Journal of Computer-Assisted Tomography, 22,* 471–479.

Schlosser, M. J., et al. (1998). Functional MRI studies of auditory comprehension. *Human Brain Mapping, 6,* 1–13.

Schmitt, J. E., Eliez, S., Bellugi, U., & Reiss, A. L. (2001). Analysis of cerebral shape in Williams syndrome. *Archives of Neurology, 58(2),* 283–287.

Schmitt, J. E., Eliez, S., Warsofsky, I., Bellugi, U., & Reiss, A. L. (2001). Corpus callosum morphology of Williams Syndrome: Relationships to genetics and behavior. *Developmental Medicine and Child Neurology, 43(3):* 155–159.

Sirevaag, A. M., Black, J. E., Shafron, D., & Greenough, W. T. (1988). Direct evidence that complex experience increases capillary branching and surface area in visual cortex of young rats. *Brain Research, 471,* 299–304.

Subramanium, B., Hennessey, J. G., Rubin, M. A., Beach, L. S., & Reiss, A. L. (1997). Software and methods for quantitative imaging in neuroscience: The Kennedy Krieger Institute Human Brain Project. In S. H. Koslow & M. F. Huerta (Eds.), *Neuroinformatics: An overview of the human brain project* (pp. 335–360). Hillsdale, NJ: Erlbaum.

Wang, J. Y., Frenzel, K. E., Wen, D., & Falls, D. L. (1998). Transmembrane neuregulins interact with LIM kinase 1, a cytoplasmic protein kinase implicated in development of visuospatial cognition. *Journal of Biological Chemistry, 273,* 20525–20534.

Wang, P. P., Hesselink, J. R., Jernigan, T. L., Doherty, S., & Bellugi, U. (1992). Specific neurobehavioral profile of Williams syndrome is associated with neocerebellar hemispheric preservation. *Neurology, 42,* 1999–2002.

Wang, Y. K., Samos, C. H., Peoples, R., Perez-Jurado, L. A., Nusse, R., & Francke, U. (1997). A novel human homologue of the Drosophila frizzled wnt receptor gene binds wingless protein and is in the Williams syndrome deletion at 7q11.23. *Human Molecular Genetics, 6,* 465–472.

Williams Syndrome Association 6th National/International Professional Conference Abstracts. (1994). *Genetic Counseling, 6,* 131–192.

Zatorre, R. J., Evans, A. C., & Meyer, E. (1994). Neural mechanisms underlying melodic perception and memory for pitch. *Journal of Neuroscience, 14,* 1908–1919.

5 Cellular and Molecular Cortical Neuroanatomy in Williams Syndrome

Albert M. Galaburda and Ursula Bellugi

The purpose of a neuroanatomical analysis of Williams Syndrome (WMS) brains is to help bridge the knowledge of the genetics of this disorder with the knowledge on behavior. Here, we outline findings of cortical neuroanatomy at multiple levels. We describe the gross anatomy with respect to brain shape, cortical folding, and asymmetry. This, as with most neuroanatomical information available in the literature on anatomical-functional correlations, links up best to the behavioral profile. Then, we describe the cytoarchitectonic appearance of the cortex. Further, we report on some histometric results. Finally, we present findings of immunocytochemistry that attempt to link up to the genomic deletion. The gross anatomical findings consist mainly of a small brain that shows curtailment in the posterior-parietal and occipital regions. There is also subtle dysmorphism of cortical folding. A consistent finding is a short central sulcus that does not become opercularized in the interhemispheric fissure, bringing attention to a possible developmental anomaly affecting the dorsal half of the hemispheres. There is also lack of asymmetry in the planum temporale. The cortical cytoarchitecture is relatively normal, with all sampled areas showing features typical of the region from which they are taken. Measurements in area 17 show increased cell size and decreased cell-packing density, which address the issue of possible abnormal connectivity. Immunostaining shows absence of elastin but normal staining for Lim-1 kinase, both of which are products of genes that are part of the deletion. Finally, one serially sectioned brain shows a fair amount of acquired pathology of microvascular origin related most likely to underlying hypertension and heart disease.

Introduction

Behavioral and Genetic Characteristics to be Explained by Neuroanatomy

Williams Syndrome (WMS) provides a unique opportunity to study the brain in a condition where the genetic basis is understood and the cognitive profile is highly distinctive and well characterized, and may represent a prototype neurocognitive disorder for the study of the relationship between genes and behavior via the uncovering of the anatomical structures that intervene. The main idea is that complex behaviors, including cognitive and emotional behaviors, are implemented in large neural systems that are formed in part from genetic blueprints and in part through learning. Moreover, the reaction of the brain to the learning environment itself is partly controlled by genes.

The field of cognitive neuroscience thus far has been able to expand our knowledge about where different neural systems are located in the brain and what types of mental activity activates or suppress these neural systems. This information, together with older information from the study of patients with neurological damage, have shown, for example, that the frontal lobes are involved in many aspects of working memory, and that the primary visual cortex participates in mental imagery. The systems in question are built from the bottom up through a sequence of timed molecular processes involving developmental genes, and the same structures are maintained and modified throughout life through the action of additional molecular events. Thus, a clinical condition affecting gene structure and function can be well placed to modify the building of cognitively relevant brain structures and their maintenance throughout life, which in turn can affect the behaviors that these structures support. Furthermore, behavior itself is capable of modifying the brain structures that support it. In this sense, the structure of the brain lies between the genes involved in their development and maintenance and the behaviors they support and by which they are modified.

Anatomy is the logical link between genes and behavior. The purpose of our research on the neuroanatomy of WMS is to help link the anatomical findings to the genetic/molecular disorder on the one hand and to the behavior disorder on the other, thus helping to link genes to cognition and emotion. Specifically, an anatomical research program in WMS must ultimately be able to explain the relationship between the deleted genes in region 7q11.23 (Perez-Jurado et al., 1998; Osborne et al., 1997a, 1997b; Wang et al., 1997; see also Korenberg et al., 1996; Korenberg et al., 1997a; Korenberg, Chen, Mitchell, & Sun, 1997b; Korenberg et al., 1998; Korenberg et al., chap. 6) and the building and maintenance of brain structures on the one hand, and, on the other hand, the abnormal behaviors, consisting of mental retardation, visuo-spatial deficits, relatively good linguistic abilities, an unusual personality, and good facial recognition and musical abilities (Jones et al., chap. 2; Lenhof, Wang, Greenberg, & Bellugi, 1997; Bellugi, Klima, & Wang, 1996; Bellugi, Adolphs, Cassady, & Chiles, 1999a; Bellugi, Lai, & Korenberg, in press; Bellugi, Lichtenberger, Mills, Galaburda, & Korenberg, 1999b; Bellugi, Mills, Jernigan, Hickok, & Galaburda, 1999c; Bellugi, Lichtenberg, Jones, Lai, & St. George, chap. 1).

Of great importance to the understanding of the general biology of WMS, are the findings of distinctive facial features and cardiovascular defects, which typically include supravalvular aortic stenosis or pulmonic stenosis, calcium metabolism abnormalities, failure to thrive in infancy, and delayed development. Genetic diagnosis is now possible, and, in almost all individuals clinically identified with WMS, it has been found that there is a hemizygous deletion of one copy of the elastin gene and adjacent genes (Lowery et al., 1995; Ewart et al., 1993). Other genes involved in the deletion, in most cases, include Lim-1 kinase, RF2c, FZD3, and syntaxin 1A (see Korenberg et al., chap. 6; Perez-Jurado et al., 1998; Osborne et al., 1997a, 1997b; Wang et al., 1997).

Just as neuroanatomy is placed somewhere between gene expression and behavior, so is neurophysiology. Some relevant neurophysiologic findings, therefore, will be reviewed. Thus, a series of studies has been undertaken using event-related potential techniques (ERPs) to assess the timing and organization of neural systems that are active during sensory, cognitive, and language processing in WMS subjects (Mills, 1998; Mills et al., chap. 3; Neville, Mills, & Bellugi, 1995). Two of the notable characteristics of the WMS behavioral profile have so far been investigated. First, the auditory recovery cycle has been tested for indices of hyperexcitability at any stage along the auditory pathway that might provide clues to the basis of the sensitivity to auditory stimuli shown by many WMS subjects. Second, auditory sentence processing, which includes semantic anomalies has been assessed as to whether such processing is mediated in WMS by the same pathways that are active in normal age-matched controls. Auditory brainstem evoked responses turn out to be normal in WMS subjects, indicating that auditory hyperexcitability does not occur at the brainstem level. However, data from an auditory recovery paradigm suggest a possible cortical mechanism; WMS subjects are indistinguishable from normal controls on a visual recovery paradigm. Taken together, these studies suggest that the hyperacusis observed in WMS may be mediated by hyperexcitability specifically within the cortical areas that are utilized in processing acoustic information. Guided by this finding, Hickok and collaborators found that Heschl's gyrus may be larger in WMS (Bellugi et al., 1999b; Hickok et al., 1995).

ERPs have also been recorded of WMS subjects' responses to auditorily presented words in sentences (Mills, Neville, Appelbaum, Prat, & Bellugi, 1997). One half of the sentences were highly contextually constrained, ending with a semantically appropriate word, whereas the other half ended with an anomalous word (e.g., "I take my coffee with cream and paper."). Previous research has shown that normal subjects indicate a large negative response at 400 msec (N400) to semantically unprimed words, and this is considered as an index of how the mental lexicon is organized. WMS subjects displayed responses that were abnormal within the first 200–300 msec following word onset. The abnormality consisted of a positivity, not seen in normal control subjects. This effect, only apparent over temporal brain regions, may relate to WMS hyperacusis. The effect of the semantic anomaly is larger over the left hemisphere in WMS than in the controls, which may be related to the unusual semantic proclivities shown by WMS subjects in certain tasks (Bellugi et al., 1996; Bellugi et al., 1999b). Moreover, the WMS responses did not show the expected left-hemisphere asymmetries for grammatical function words that are typical for normal children and adults, suggesting that there may be an unusual pattern of brain organization underlying the WMS language capacities.

From the point of view of the neuroanatomy of WMS, these behavioral characteristics conjure up a variety of dichotomies: (1) Involvement of parietal vs. frontal areas; (2) Involvement of right-hemisphere vs. left-hemisphere structures; (3) Involvement of dorsal streams (sometimes clumped together with magnocellular streams [see Atkinson et al., 1997], as opposed to the ventral [parvocellular] streams) and, finally, (4) Involvement of cortical vs. subcortical anatomical systems.

New techniques of brain imaging permit visualization and analysis of structures within the brain that were not possible in the past. Techniques developed, e.g., by Frank, Damasio, and Grabowski (1997) (also, see Reiss et al., chap. 4), now permit an unprecedented visualization and three-dimensional analysis of the living brain of subjects. Initial studies revealed that both WMS and DNS leave a distinctive morphological stamp on specific brain regions. Past MRI studies of brain volumes were performed on a group of matched adolescents and young adults with WMS and DNS (Bellugi, Hickok, Lai, & Jernigan, 1997; Jernigan & Bellugi, 1990, 1994). Neuromorphological characterization of WMS vs. DNS subjects by magnetic resonance imaging showed that the cerebral volume in both groups was smaller than that of age-matched normal controls. Analyses revealed important regional differences in brain volume between the two groups of subjects. First, anterior-brain volume was found to be disproportionately reduced in DNS subjects but proportionately preserved in subjects with WMS. Secondly, limbic structures in the temporal lobe showed essentially equal volumes in WMS and control subjects, but were significantly reduced in DNS subjects. On the other hand, the volume of the thalamus and lenticular nuclei were seen to be much better preserved in subjects with DNS than those with WMS. We also found that the anterior parts of the corpus callosum, like the anterior hemispheres, were preserved in WMS subjects, but diminished in DNS subjects (Wang, Doherty, Hesselink, & Bellugi, 1992).

Quantitative analysis of cerebellar volumes also suggested differences with cerebellar volume well preserved in WMS subjects but diminished in DNS subjects. Closer regional analyses were enlightening: Jernigan and Bellugi (1994) found that the locus of preservation in WMS was the neocerebellum. Of the two parts of the neocerebellum that were subjected to analysis, the neocerebellar vermis and the neocerebellar tonsils both showed volumetric preservation or even *increases* in WMS as compared to controls, whereas, both were found to be volumetrically diminished in DNS. Importantly, the specific regions of the neocerebellum that may be enlarged in WMS were shown to be dysplagic in autism (Jones, Lai, & Bellugi, 1999; Jernigan, Wang, & Bellugi, 1995; Courchesne, Yeung-Courchesne, Press, Hesselink, & Jernigan, 1988; Courchesne, Bellugi, & Singer, 1995).

More recently, Reiss et al. (chap. 4) carried out MRI studies with higher resolution techniques. In 14 young adult subjects with WMS and an aged-matched control group, the decreased in total brain volume was confirmed, as well as the relative preservation of the cerebellum. The superior-temporal gyrus was also found to be relatively preserved, an area that contains the auditory system and those auditory association areas that form part of language networks. There was also a significant curtailment of the volume of the brainstem. A greater ratio of frontal to parieto-occipital forebrain volume was also found, and there was reduction of the forebrain white matter, with relative preservation of the cerebrocortical volume. Nonetheless, regionally, the right-occipital lobe showed excessive volume loss.

Results of related research suggest that the expansive prefrontal cortex and the neocerebellum, both selectively (relatively) preserved in WMS, are thought to be closely related. These two regions of the brain are most highly developed in *Homo sapiens,* and are thought to have evolved contemporaneously (Deacon, 1990). Furthermore, the neocerebellum has more extensive connections to prefrontal and other association areas of the cortex than do the older parts of the cerebellum. On the other hand, the reduction in the forebrain white matter may explain the curtailment of the brainstem, but it may be relevant to note that FZD3, which is one of the deleted genes, is associated with hindbrain segmentation, which could also explain, in part, the brainstem changes in WMS. Thus, the neuroanatomic profile of WMS emerging from neuroimaging is beginning to contribute to the understanding of the brain's organization by exhibiting a morphological pattern that can result from genetic bias. The finding that frontal and neocerebellar regions are selectively preserved in WMS suggests that they all may come under the influence of a single genetic, developmental factor, or that their development is mutually interactive, or both (Bellugi et al., 1999c). These issues bearing on the relationship of brain to behavior are fundamental to central questions of cognitive neuroscience.

Results

Gross Anatomical Observations on Autopsy Specimens

The findings reported below are based on the study of four WMS brains from patients diagnosed in life on the basis of the typical somatic phenotype as well as genetic testing. The gross anatomical findings may be summarized as follows.

Brain Weight and Shape   Brain weight and shape are variable, but mostly we have seen small brains with parietal and occipital hypoplasia (Figure 5.1). The brain weight hovers around 800–1000 g, which is roughly in the order of the brain weights of patients with DNS. The shape, however, is different. In DNS, there is an antero-posterior curtailment of the brain, whereas this brachycephaly is not seen in WMS. Instead, the

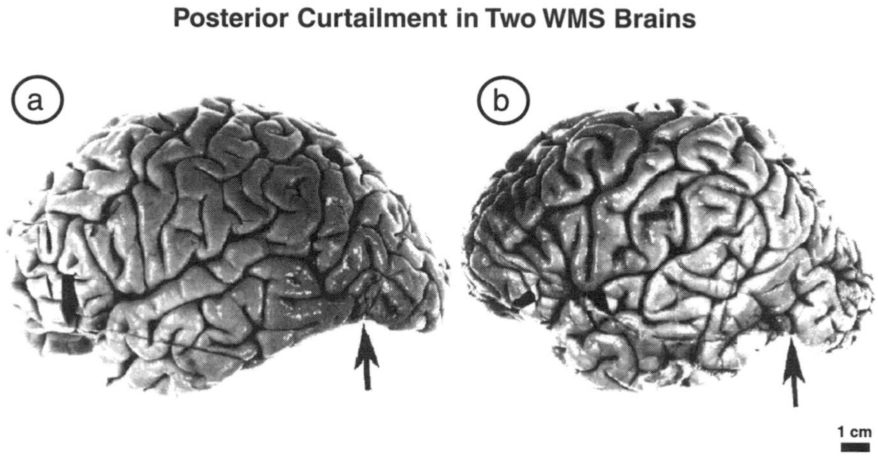

Posterior Curtailment in Two WMS Brains

Figure 5.1
The arrows point to a marked indentation of the temporoparietal region in the area of the temporoparietal sulcus. However, note that the whole posterior-parietal and occipital regions are small.

brain appears rather curtailed from top to bottom, especially in the posterior portions of the hemispheres. One of the specimens that we examined showed a striking top to bottom curtailment of the occipito-parietal regions on both hemispheres (Galaburda, Wang, Bellugi, & Rossen, 1994), which was not observed in the other three specimens, at least not to the same degree; but see Figure 5.1, which shows a clear but less dramatic curtailment in two specimens. There may also be modifications of the standard patterns of brain asymmetry that involve the planum temporale and the occipital lobe.

Cortical Folding and Asymmetry   We have looked for anomalous gyri and found these to be variable. There is, however, a frequent finding of anomalous sulci in the dorso-medial portions of the hemispheres. A consistent finding in all four cases studied is made in the central sulcus. Unlike control brains, where the central sulcus reaches the interhemispheric fissure and proceeds a variable distance along the medial surface of the hemisphere in a characteristic posteriorly curved direction, the central sulcus in the WMS brains ends substantially before it reaches the midline (Figure 5.2). We are now looking at this region in larger numbers of WMS subjects on MRI images in collaboration with Allan Reiss (Reiss et al., chap. 4).

Reduced Volume of Amygdala   We were able to examine one of the specimens for morphology of the amygdalar nuclei. The overall volume of the amygdala was diminished in the WMS specimen, and was estimated to be about half the size of the average amygdala in controls. Also, note that the temporal horn (TH) is more dorsally placed in

Foreshortened Central Sulci, Particularly in the Dorso-Medial Portions in WMS

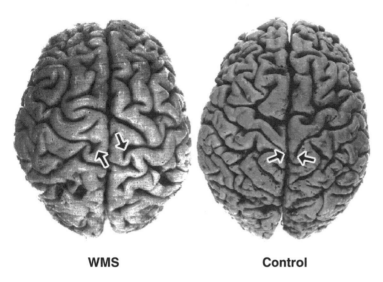

WMS   **Control**

Figure 5.2
Note the difference in the medial reach (arrows) of the central sulci between the WMS and Control subjects, particularly in the dorsomedial portions of the hemispheres.

WMS. Furthermore, there was an unusual scooping out of the nucleus in the region of the dorsal portion of the lateral subnucleus of the amygdala. This nucleus receives connections from visual association cortex (Figure 5.3). Of course, it would be premature to make too much of this finding in a single brain. However, if the finding is consistent among WMS brains, one would be prone to attempt a connection between this finding and the lack of stranger shyness in this group also characterized as hypersociability (Jones et al., this volume; Bellugi et al., 1999a). Thus, if visual and auditory experience does not acquire the proper emotional valence via the amygdalar circuit, the ancient way to avoid danger may be lost (Damasio, 1994).

Parenchymal Softenings, Meningeal, Vascular, and Other Neuropathological Findings Notably Absent   In view of the commonly found cardiac and vascular pathology in WMS, we searched for evidence of vascular injury to the brain, presumably acquired during life and not resulting directly from genetic errors. We found none. In general, the cortex was intact, the blood vessels at the base of the brain and on the convexity were normal for age, and the meninges showed no evidence of previous bleeding.

Reduced Volume of Amygdala in WMS

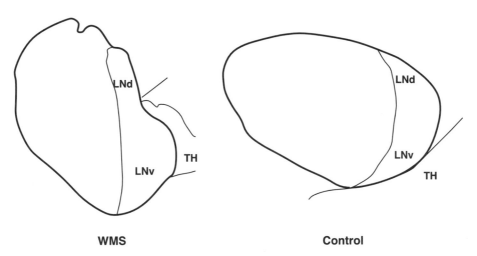

WMS   **Control**

Figure 5.3
Amygdalar nuclei in WMS and normal brains, showing that in WMS the dorsal portion of the lateral nucleus (LNd) appears to be reduced and has an unusual shape. The arrow indicates a curtailment in the lateral nucleus of the amygdala. In this specimen, the nucleus was estimated to be about half the size of the average amygdala in normal subjects. Also, note that in the temporal horn (TH) is placed more dorsally in WMS individuals than in normal subjects.

Architectonic Observations

We examined blocks of tissue selected from most classes of cortex for architectonic differentiation. The architectonic level of analysis refers to the anatomical level smaller that gyri and sulci (gross), but larger than the level of single cells (histological). This level permits analysis of the laminar and columnar arrangement of neurons and glia, myelin content, and vascularization, which under normal conditions shows remarkable regional differentiation based on proportions of large and small neurons, thickness of layers, presence or absence of columns, and other related features. This level of analysis has led to cortical architectonic maps such as those of Brodmann, von Economo and Koskinas, and others. The architectonic differentiation reflects, in part, cortical differentiation in connectivity and physiological properties of individual neurons comprising the areas. The architectonic findings may be summarized as follows.

Areas All areas sampled appeared relatively normal and recognizable according to established criteria for identification of architectonic areas. Thus, we noted well-differentiated primary cortices such as areas 4, 17, and 42, visual and auditory, respectively, first belt of association cortices such as areas 6, 18, and 22, and so-called integration or high-order association cortices, such as areas 37, 39, and 9 (all listed in the Brodmann nomenclature). This is compatible with the finding of relatively normal gyral folding, which reflects at least in part architectonic differentiation of the cortex.

Increased Cell-Packing Density in Cortex   We noted a tendency, albeit not uniform, for the cortex to show increased cell-packing density, coarseness of neurons, and mild dysplastic features (Galaburda et al., 1994)—but see the histometric studies below for a more detailed analysis.

No Systematic Bias Affecting Architecture   In view of the question regarding the intactness or lack thereof of the dorsoventral (magnocellular/parvocellular) dichotomy (see above), we looked for a systematic bias possibly affecting the architecture of dorsal parietal regions. We found none. There were also no other biases (e.g., frontal vs. parietal, left vs. right hemisphere). We cannot comment on the cortical vs. subcortical dichotomy based on the available material, including the amygdala.

One of our autopsy cases was processed in whole-brain coronal sections rather than in blocks of tissue, thus allowing a more thorough survey of the architectonic areas. While surveying this case, we noted neuropathological changes not of the developmental, but rather of the acquired cortical injury type, which had not been evident on the gross examination of this brain (see above). Thus, we saw evidence of microvascular pathology affecting the cortex of predominantly the dorsal hemispheres, parietal more than frontal (Figure 5.4). These consisted of gliotic small infarcts within the cortical ribbon and outside in the cortical subcortical junction. All of these lesions were well healed and could not be dated other than to say that they were at least a few months old. Stains for myelin

Microvascular Lesions in WMS, Primarily in Dorsal, Parietal, and Occipital Lobes

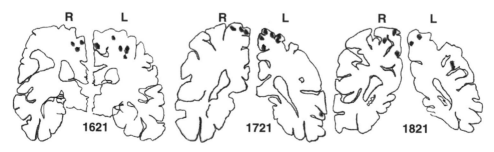

Figure 5.4
Serial sections taken from WMS-3 showing microvascular lesions mainly in the dorsal-parietal and occipital lobes. Numbers refer to the section number; R = right hemisphere; L = left hemisphere.

aimed at determining whether the lesions leading to these scars took place within the first year or two of life were negative, thus indicating that the injury was not likely to have been perinatal. However, the location of these scars with respect to the dorsal-ventral dichotomy raised questions as to their connection with the behavioral profile of patients with WMS. For one, it raised the previously not considered possibility that the cognitive profile might also be related to acquired as well as genetic brain abnormalities.

Histometric Observations

At the level of histological analysis, that is, of single neurons, as at higher and lower levels, it is possible also to make quantitative statements such as density and size of neurons (histometric). This is an important step beyond architectonic analysis to document and expand on information gleaned at that level as well as for search for subtler changes that may not be obvious at the architectonic level. For instance, changes in the number of neurons have implications regarding generation of neurons and apoptosis, while changes in neuronal size make statements about neuronal connectivity. We are currently carrying out an extensive histometric analysis of theoretically relevant architectonic areas in WMS. The goal of the study is to compare histometric changes, if any, between areas in the dorsal and ventral forebrain, in keeping with the hypothesis that these two cortical regions will be differentially affected by the deletion.

The primary visual cortex Brodmann area 17 (also primary visual cortex, V1), is easily identified under low power microscopy based on the unique tripartite appearance of layer IV (IV a, b, and c, with the latter further subdivided into IVcα and β. Blocks of calcarine cortex were taken from the middle portion of the calcarine fissure, which represents peripheral vision and projects heavily to the dorsal visual pathways. Layers II, III, IVa, IVb, IVcα, IVcβ, V, and VI of area 17 were measured in each hemisphere. We used ANOVA to determine cell-packing density (CPD) and neuronal size differences between the WMS and control cases. The independent measures included diagnosis (WMS and control), hemisphere (right and left), and layer (II, III, IVa, IVb, IVcα, IVcβ, V, and VI). The dependent measures were cell size and cell-packing density. The effect of gender could not be analyzed with any confidence because of the small number of cases. Neuronal size distributions were analyzed using Chi-square tests.

There was a layer by diagnosis interaction in the left hemisphere in cell-packing density, and WMS brains had greater packing of neurons in layer IVcβ in the left hemisphere (see Figure 5.5). Further, there was an hemispheric asymmetry in cell-packing density in favor of the left hemisphere in layer III in WMS but not in controls. Together, with these changes in cell-packing density there was a difference in the proportion of neuronal sizes between control and WMS brains, whereby WMS brains had an excess of small neurons and a paucity of large neurons by comparison to control brains in granular and infragranular layers, which was due to effects of the left hemisphere (see Figure 5.6).

Neuronal Density in Left Primary Visual Cortex

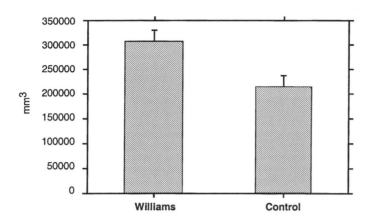

Figure 5.5
Neuronal packing density difference between WMS and age- and sex-matched control brains in layer IVcβ of a part of visual area 17 subserving peripheral retina.

Distribution of Neuronal Size in Left Primary Visual Cortex

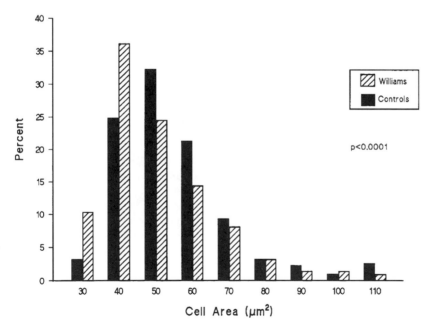

Figure 5.6
Difference in the distribution of neuronal sizes between WMS and age- and sex-matched control brains in layer IVcβ of a part of visual area 17 subserving peripheral retina. WMS has more small cells and fewer larger cells than controls.

Also, subtle changes in hemispheric parameters between WMS and control brains support demonstrated differences in cerebral lateralization in WMS. Thus, an area of the visual cortex related to the dorsal visual pathway shows histometric differences in WMS as compared to control brains. These changes are compatible with smaller, more highly packed neurons in a smaller brain, rather than a change in neuronal numbers, which in turn are more readily explained by changes in connectivity in WMS rather than by alterations in generation and/or loss of neurons. It remains to be seen whether these types of changes affect cortex representing central vision too, or whether the changes are of a different type.

Molecular Observations

As genes relating to the WMS deletions are just being discovered, it has been difficult to obtain specific antibodies and mRNA probes that react with human autopsy tissue. It is also worth remembering that with a hemi-deletion, the assumption, unless the function of the remaining allele is removed through imprinting, is that some gene function remains. In some cases, this gene function may be sufficient to code for detectable product. In others, there may be a threshold effect, with an all-or-none behavior. Barring technical problems, which abound in this area of research, lack of staining indicates that no gene function exists, whereas, positive staining does not address the issue of quantitative adequacy of gene function. The findings thus far, however, may be summarized as follows.

Elastin   Elastin does not stain in forebrain neurons or glia, and is only found in blood vessels and meninges in normal forebrain. In the cerebellum, however, elastin stains normally in Purkinje cells and in mouse elastin messenger RNA is demonstrated in Purkinje neurons by in situ hybridization (Sawchenko, Dargusch, Arias, & Bellugi, 1997). The normal control cerebellum showed the immunostaining for elastin in Purkinje neurons, whereas the WMS brain did not (Figure 5.7).

Lim-1 Kinase   Lim-1 kinase appears to stain many forebrain neurons in normal human brain. Likewise, and unlike elastin, there is probably normal staining for Lim-1 kinase in the WMS cerebral cortex (Figure 5.8).

Detailed Studies

Of the four WMS brain specimens, only one was processed in whole-brain serial sections and all are blocked for architectonic analysis. Blocks were taken of the dorsolateral- and ventrolateral-prefrontal cortex, superior- and inferior-parietal lobules, dorsal- and ventral-preoccipital cortex, superior-temporal gyrus, Heschl's auditory gyrus, and calcarine cortex. The blocks were embedded in celloidin, which provides the best medium for Nissl staining. Nissl staining was accomplished with cresyl violet,

Elastin Staining in Cerebellar Purkinje Cells in Normals and WMS

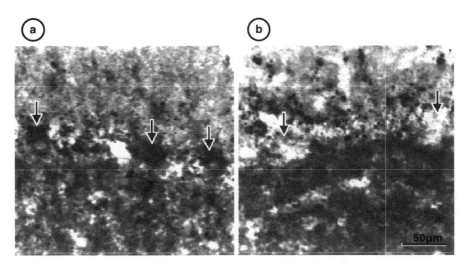

Figure 5.7
(a) Cerebellar Purkinje cells showing positive immunostaining for elastin Normals (arrows); (b) Arrows point to areas occupied by Purkinje cells in WMS-1, which do not stain for elastin.

Lim-1 Kinase Staining in WMS

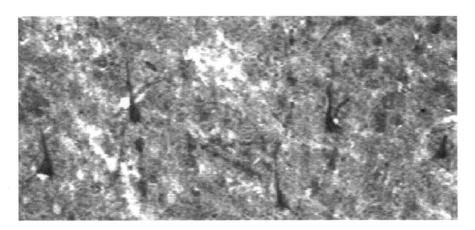

Figure 5.8
Immunostain disclosing positive neurons in the cerebral cortex of WMS for Lim-1 kinase. This is a hemideleted gene that still expresses in WMS-3 in contrast to elastin, which does not (see Figure 5.7 for comparison).

which endows the cells with a purplish blue color of uniform intensity and suitable for histometric studies (see below). The architecture of a given region is analyzed under low power light microscopy with regards to several classic architectonic parameters: Overall cortical thickness, relative thickness of the laminae, impression of the cell-packing density of the cortex as a whole, general comparisons in this parameter between supra- and infra-granular layers, and the cell-packing density (CPD) of individual layers, a sense of coarseness or fineness of the cellular panorama, which is determined by the relative sizes of the neurons comprising the layers, the way in which one layer is defined from its neighbors or melds with them, the way in which layer 6 neurons border with the subcortical white matter.

The prefrontal cortices are relatively thick, relatively sparsely celled, but more densely packed in the infra- than in the supra-granular layers, containing relatively coarse pyramidal neurons. Although the granule cell layers are evident, they are never as richly packed as in the more posterior cortices of the temporal and parietal lobes. Laminar distinctiveness is not nearly as explicit as in the parietal cortices, and this is particularly true in the inferior-prefrontal cortices, which are more granular than the dorsal-prefrontal cortex, and where the granular layers blur the borders among the adjacent layers. All of these features are well developed in the frontal cortices in WMS. In general, there is the impression of increased cell-packing density, a feature that has been reported by us previously. As will be seen below when the histomorphometric findings are reported and discussed, it turns out that this impression of increased cell-packing density is the result of increased glial cells, which under the low-power magnification used for architectonic analysis cannot be distinguished from small granular neurons. In the brain processed in serial histological sections, a previously unpredicted set of abnormalities was seen in the frontal lobe, which will be discussed below.

The parietal cortices are the most distinctively laminated in the brain, short of the primary visual cortex, and the dorsal-parietal cortex is even more so because of their relative hypogranularity compared to the ventral-parietal cortices. Granular neurons in layers 2 and 4 tend to blur laminar borders and render the overall impression of the cortex less laminated. Furthermore, the dorsal-parietal cortices show a distinct clearing of the region deep to layer 3c, adding to the layered appearance of the cortex. In general, because of decreased granularity and coarser pyramidal neurons, the dorsal-parietal cortices are coarser than the cortices of the inferior-parietal lobule. Special attention was paid to the architecture of the dorsal-parietal cortices in WMS, because this area is implicated in the behavioral abnormalities, either because of its contribution to the magno-cellular visual system, or because of its known role in the performance of visuo-spatial tasks. However, no obvious architectonic distortion could be seen in these areas in WMS other than those that appear to characterize the cortex of WMS in general: An impression of increased cell-packing density and greater coarseness of the cellular architecture. In the frontal lobe, where the cortex is naturally coarse, this feature was less obvious; but, in the parietal cortex, the coarseness in WMS is more easily perceived under low-power magnification. In the brain processed in serial histological sections, a previously unpredicted set of abnormalities was seen in the parietal lobe, which will be discussed below.

The occipital cortices are similar in appearance to the parietal cortices, except for the primary visual cortex, area 17, which contains a highly differentiated layer 4 with three sublaminae—a, b, and c (a and b). The temporal cortices also resemble the parietal cortices in that layer 4 is well formed. There are differences between the cortical areas covering the superior and the middle- and inferior-temporal gyri, with the latter having a more ribbon-like appearance of layer 4, and the former being among the more granular of all sensory related cortices. The WMS cortical areas were examined with the above criteria in mind, and no significant abnormalities are noted in any of the samples taken.

Case Studies   Our first case was a patient with WMS who died of cardiac complications of the disease at age 31 years (see Galaburda et al., 1994). The gross morphology of the brain was abnormal in that the parietal regions are reduced dramatically in size in comparison to the frontal regions, a finding that did not reproduce in any of the following cases to the same degree. The presplenial portion of the corpus callosum was thinned, as was the case in WMS-2–94, but not so in the other two cases. Cytoarchitectonic abnormalities were found throughout the cortex and consisted of primitive layering similar to that found in brains 1–2 years of age; these, however, were subtle in nature, and the normal variability in this feature is not well understood. Histological findings were of two types: There was increased cell-packing density, as compared to an age-matched control brain; neurons were often found in clusters in abnormal position and location, including excessive Cajal-Retzius cells in the molecular layer and clusters of subcortical neurons. The capillaries of the cortex displayed a primitive morphology, and we saw several subcortical arterioles surrounded by inflammatory cells. Areas of abnormal gyral formation did not show especially different microscopic anomalies, and in this one specimen, we could not ascertain a rostro-caudal gradient in malformation to match the gross anatomical finding of relative sparing of the frontal portions of the forebrain. We searched for, but did not find, nodular heterotopias, microgyria, pachygyria, porencephaly, ulegyria, or other similarly severe examples of developmental malformation.

Our second case was that of an 8-month-old baby who died of SIDS. The brain was harvested fresh rather than fixed. The gyral pattern appeared normal, but in retrospect, the dorsomedial portions of the hemispheres may be abnormal. The presplenial area of the corpus callosum was thinned, as in the other case. Some of the histological sections are examined and showed increased cell-packing density, although controls in this age group still need to be examined. Immunostains for AchE, CAT-301, laminin, CGRP, and elastin were run. AchE and laminin stained well. CGRP may be expressed excessively, but this needs confirmation against age-matched controls. CAT-301, which relates mostly to the magnocellular visual pathway, is found normally. Elastin did not stain in this brain. In an older control brain, elastin was seen in blood vessel walls (the tropoelastin form present intracellularly). The significance of these findings awaits stains of control tissue.

Our third case was that of a 53-year-old woman who died of cardiac failure. The diagnosis of WMS was not made until she was 39 years of age, but was extensively tested by our collaborators at The Salk Institute. A general postmortem examination was not done, but the brain was donated directly to this laboratory. The brain weight was 900 g, which is small. The cortical folding appeared normal, and there was lack of asymmetry of the planum temporale as well as reversed petalia in the frontal and occipital ends. Cytoarchitecture was normal, without apparent increase in cell-packing density, but still showing somewhat coarse neurons. Again, the architecture of representative areas of the frontal, parietal, occipital, and temporal lobes was basically normal in that no areas are found to be missing and the appearance of the areas was standard according to cytoarchitectonic criteria. However, this method allowed for the discovery of an unpredicted finding: There was evidence throughout the telencephalon, but most strikingly in the dorsal portions of the hemispheres, and more so in the parietal than in the frontal cortices, of a multiplicity of microvascular infarcts with gliosis and neuronal loss (see Figure 5.4). There had been no history of strokes during life, but we would suggest that the heart disease that is part of WMS may be associated with showers of emboli that produce microinfarcts in the dorsal borderzone vascular territories. Of importance to the present research is the realization that at least, in part, the behavioral picture in WMS may be the result of acquired brain damage through vascular injury and not only the genetic defect. Certainly, the predominant involvement of the dorsal portions of the brain, back more so than front, is compatible with a behavioral profile of visuo-spatial dysfunction and attentional deficits, with sparing of facial recognition and language. Unfortunately, the only certain way to check whether this finding is consistent across cases is by whole-brain serial section processing, which is expensive and time-consuming. We are also looking for ways by which the pathology described above can be demonstrated by magnetic resonance imaging during life, but this appears unlikely by virtue of the small size of the individual infarcts and their presence almost entirely intracortically, where imaging artifacts are more common and issues of contrast sensitivity play a larger role in visualization.

An important caveat of the interpretation that the acquired cortical lesions in this case may be related to the apparently dorsal parieto-occipital profile of WMS cognitive dysfunction, is the possibility that the vascular pathology may exist without the cognitive profile. This is because it appears to be the case that individuals with just the elastin gene deletion, who have heart disease but no cognitive defects, are equally likely to have the embolic disorder. It is still possible, however, that the behavioral picture is the result of a combination of acquired and developmental changes in the brain, and that either alone may produce a much more subtle clinical picture. We are of course interested in processing a brain of pure elastin gene deletion from a behaviorally tested subject to expand our knowledge on this question, but admittedly this specimen will be difficult to locate.

Our fourth case came from a 46-year-old woman who died of metastatic breast carcinoma. During life, her brain had been imaged by our collaborators at The Salk Institute. The fixed brain was small, weighing only 1000 g. The cortical folding was relatively normal, but for bilaterally small superior-parietal lobules, symmetry of the planum temporale, and reversed frontal petalia. As with the other cases, there was the abnormal morphology of the superior-central region and the short central sulcus bilaterally. The cytoarchitecture of the selected blocks was normal, except for the appearance of increased cell-packing density and somewhat coarse neurons. The brain was chosen for histometric analysis because of the availability of an age- and gender-matched control. The results of the histometric analysis are presented above. In addition (see Figures 5.7 and 5.8), brain sections were immunostained for elastin and Lim-1 kinase. Whereas the latter was demonstrated in forebrain cortical neurons, elastin did not stain in WMS cerebellum but did stain in control Purkinje neurons.

Histomorphometric Results   Results are available for two WMS and two control brains in the primary visual cortex. Several hundred neurons were measured and counted in each specimen under $40 \times$ oil-immersion magnification with the aid of a computer-assisted morphometric analysis system. Cells are counted inside optical boxes, which provides a reliable measure of cell-packing density. Cell-packing density does not directly address the question of cell numbers. In general, with a brain of equivalent size, increased cell-packing density would indicate increased numbers of neurons and vice versa. With a smaller brain, which is the case in WMS, increased cell-packing density could signify increased numbers of neurons, no change in the number of neurons, or even decreased numbers of neurons depending on how much smaller the brain is and how much greater the cell-packing density. Decreased cell-packing density or no change in cell-packing density from controls, in WMS, would definitely indicate smaller numbers of neurons overall. It should be noted that three out of the four WMS brains examined under low-power light microscopy for cytoarchitectonics showed what appeared to be increased cell-packing density. This finding has not been confirmed in the histomorphometric analysis, thus far. In fact, if anything, the cell-packing density is diminished in WMS. We can account for this by the observation that glial nuclei cannot be distinguished from small granular neurons under the low-power microscopy needed for cytoarchitectonics. However, under oil immersion, this distinction is easy and many of the cells that may have contributed to the impression of high cell-packing density under low power turned out to be glia instead. This finding illustrates the need to carry out high-magnification histometric analysis and the value of multi-level neuroanatomical study. If additional studies confirm the finding of lowered cell-packing density in WMS, this, coupled with a smaller brain, would indicate that the total number of neurons is decreased in WMS. This finding has been partially confirmed in the histomorphometric analysis. The finding of smaller neurons and increased packing of neurons would suggest a changed pattern of connectivity. In general, the prediction would be that there are fewer connections associated with small, packed neurons.

Molecular events observed through immunostaining for specific gene products showed that all antibodies assayed for—including laminin, acetylcholinesterase, the CAT-301 marker for the magnocellular visual pathway, and CGRP—reacted positively to the antibodies. A monoclonal antibody to tropoelastin, the intracellular form of elastin, was applied to the forebrain and cerebellum. Elastin in the forebrain was only demonstrated in blood vessels. On the other hand, Purkinje neurons are stained by the monoclonal antibody to elastin in control but not WMS cerebella. This is in spite of the fact that the deletion is hemizygous, such that there might be some production of tropoelastin. At this point, it appears that there is a threshold effect, which is not reached by virtue of the existence of the hemideletion. On the other hand, we have been able to stain WMS brain with an antibody for Lim-1 kinase, which is another gene known to be part of the hemideletion. The immunostain demonstrates cortical neurons in the forebrain, and both WMS and control brains show rich staining. Regarding elastin staining, it is thought that this matrix protein may alter neuronogenesis and neurite growth in developing brain. Elastin does not appear in glia or neurons of the forebrain in the mature state. On the other hand, elastin could be present in the matrix of forebrain structures during critical developmental periods, which has not been studied so far. Elastin is expressed in adult cerebellar Purkinje cells, and its absence in WMS may help predict for (1) local cerebellar changes in WMS and (2) alteration of fronto-cerebellar circuitries involved in behaviors such as language, motor control, and eye movements. Future research will be aimed at examining the distribution of elastin related changes in cerebellum and in forebrain areas connected with these cerebellar regions. If materials become available, additional observations may be made during development of fronto-cerebellar connections.

Ongoing work addresses expression of RF2c, FZD3, so-called "frizzled" gene, and syntaxin 1A, which are also included in the deletion. In view of the findings described thus far, it will be important not only to specify activity or lack thereof of these molecules in WMS tissue, but also to discover regional difference in expression between dorsal and ventral forebrain structures, frontal and parieto-occipital regions. An additional contrast between cortical and subcortical expression, with attention paid to the amygdala, is also important to search for.

Summary

The most consistent gross neuroanatomical finding is the abnormal length of the central sulcus, whereby the fissure does not follow its normal course dorso-medial to end on the interhemispheric surface of the hemisphere, but rather ends short 1 or 2 cm lateral to the interhemispheric fissure. This produces an unusual configuration of the dorsal central region, including the dorsal portions of the superior parietal lobule and the dorsal frontal gyrus. Of interest is the fact that it is exactly these regions that are implicated in the abnormal behavior demonstrated by patients with WMS. It should be added that the gyral markings are inconsistently anomalous, often demonstrating unusual number and configuration of gyri on the medial posterior surface of the hemispheres and on the temporal lobes. One case, that of an 11-month-old male, showed clumps of anomalous gyri giving the impression of micropolygyria (but not showing the architectonic changes associated with that malformation). Finally, there is a suggestion that brain asymmetry, as far as the planum temporale and lobar petalias, may be anomalous in this condition.

The cytoarchitecture of the cortical areas comprising the WMS forebrain appears to be mostly normal, with some differences in size of cortical neurons and packing density. Subtle dysplastic changes have been noted, which, however, are not easily quantifiable or compared to control brains. An impression of increased cell-packing density under low-power magnification turned out to be confirmed in a study of the peripheral retinal representation of the primary visual cortex affecting some layers in the left hemisphere. An additional morphometric finding was that the average size of cortical neurons in layers with increased packing density, as measured in area 17, was smaller in WMS than in control brains. These changes are compatible with changes in connectivity, but the exact extent and full interpretation await further results.

Acquired neuropathologic findings are seen in one of the cases, which was processed in whole-brain serial sections. These are consistent with microinfarcts—probably reflecting underlying heart disease and embolus formation—and affected dorsal portions of the hemispheres. The affected areas are known to mediate visuo-spatial and attentional tasks. Finally, the products of some of the deleted genes have been screened for in WMS. Elastin does not stain in the cerebellum in WMS, despite the preservation of one elastin gene in the hemideletion. Lim-1 kinase, on the other hand, another hemideleted gene, stains normally in cortical neurons in WMS.

Conclusions

The link between anatomy and behavior appears to fit a dorso-ventral (magno-parvo) dichotomy, rather than a fronto-caudal, left-right, or even a cortico-subcortical dichotomy. It is hypothesized that further analysis of MRI data with this idea in mind will disclose particular involvement of the dorsal portions of the hemispheres, both frontal and parieto-occipital. The behavioral profile indicates preservation of some but not all language functions, compatible with perisylvian language areas, which belong to the ventral system. Likewise, not all visual functions are impaired, with striking preservation of face recognition, a ventral function, in the face of striking visuo-spatial impairment, a dorsal function. Of additional interest is the possible involvement of the amygdalar visually related lateral nucleus, which may explain the lack of appropriate fear associated with new faces, even potentially threatening faces, in these subjects. Since this portion of the amygdala also receives auditory projections, one could predict that the WMS subjects may not be normally sensitive to threatening voice and speech. Conversely, the changes in social behavior may reflect abnormal on-off responses to social stimuli on the basis of cingulate cortex (dorsal frontal pathway) dysfunction.

Although the link to the genes from the anatomy is incomplete, it is amenable to discovery as more genes with brain developmental effects are identified in the deletion. The trick is to be certain that the functional integrity or absence thereof is demonstrable during early development, at a time when the neural systems are being built, and that the purported dysfunction remains and interferes with further neural plasticity during learning and growth. Moreover, even stronger support of the dorso-ventral hypothesis will be obtained if we are able to show that at least at some point during development, the affected genes are expressed more or less in the dorsal than in the ventral regions of the brain. The demonstration that one or more genes involved in the hemideletion are expressed in dorsal regions and not in ventral regions, and maintain expression throughout life, will go a long way in helping establish a link between behavior and genes in WMS. During the course of discovery, however, other, perhaps more interesting possibilities may become evident.

Notes

The research was supported by a grant from the National Institute of Child Health and Human Development (PO1 HD33113 to U. Bellugi). The authors thank the regional and national Williams Syndrome Associations and the families who assisted with these studies.

Illustrations and quotes not to be used without written permission from the author. Copyright Dr. Albert M. Galaburda, Boston, MA.

References

Atkinson, J., King, J., Braddick, O., Nokes, L., Anker, S., & Braddick, F. (1997). A specific deficit of dorsal stream function in Williams syndrome. *NeuroReport, 8,* 1919–1922.

Bellugi, U., Adolphs, R., Cassady, C., & Chiles, M. (1999a). An experimental investigation of hypersociability in Williams syndrome. *NeuroReport, 10,* 1–5.

Bellugi, U., Hickok, G., Lai, Z. C., & Jernigan, T. (1997). Links between brain & behavior: Clues to the neurobiology of Williams syndrome. *International Behavioral Neuroscience Society Abstracts, 6,* 57.

Bellugi, U., Klima, E. S., & Wang, P. P. (1996). Cognitive and neural development: Clues from genetically based syndromes. In D. Magnussen (Ed.), *The life-span development of individuals: Behavioral, neurobiological, and psychosocial perspectives* (pp. 223–243). The Nobel Symposium. New York: Cambridge University Press.

Bellugi, U., Lai, Z. C., & Korenberg, J. (In press). Genes, brains and behavior: What genetic disorders reveal about behavior. In E. Bizzi, P. Calissano, & V. Volterra (Eds.), *Frontiers of Biology Vol 4: The Brain of Homo Sapiens.* Rome, Italy: Istituto della Enciclopedia Italiana.

Bellugi, U., Lichtenberger, L., Jones, W., Lai, Z., & St. George, M. (chap. 1). The neurocognitive profile of Williams Syndrome: A complex pattern of strengths and weaknesses.

Bellugi, U., Lichtenberger, L., Mills, D., Galaburda, A., & Korenberg, J. R. (1999b). Bridging cognition, the brain and molecular genetics: Evidence from Williams syndrome. *Trends in Neurosciences, 5,* 197–207.

Bellugi, U., Mills, D., Jernigan, T., Hickok, G., & Galaburda, A. (1999c). Linking cognition, brain structure and brain function in Williams syndrome. In H. Tager-Flusberg (Ed.), *Neurodevelopmental disorders: Contributions to a new framework from the cognitive neurosciences* (pp. 111–139). Cambridge, MA: MIT Press.

Courchesne, E., Bellugi, U., & Singer, N. (1995). Infantile autism and Williams syndrome: Social and neural worlds apart. Special Issue, *Genetic Counseling, 6,* 144–145.

Courchesne, E., Yeung-Courchesne, R., Press, G. A., Hesselink, J. R., Jernigan, T. L. (1988). Hypoplasia of cerebellar vermal lobules VI and VII in autism. *New England Journal of Medicine, 318,* 1349–1354.

Damasio, A. R. (1994). *Descartes' error: Emotion, reason, and the human brain.* New York: G. P. Putnam's Sons.

Deacon, T. W. (1990). Rethinking mammalian brain evolution. *American Zoology, 30,* 629–705.

Ewart, A. K., Morris, C. A., Atkinson, D., Jin, W., Sternes, K., Spallone, P., Stock, A. D., Leppert, M., & Keating, M. T. (1993). Hemizygosity at the elastin locus in the developmental disorder, Williams syndrome. *Nature Genetics, 5,* 11–18.

Frank, R. J., Damasio, H., & Grabowski, T. J. (1997). Brainvox: An interactive, multimodal visualization and analysis system for neuroanatomical imaging. *Neuroimage, 5,* 13–30.

Galaburda, A., Wang, P. P., Bellugi, U., & Rossen, M. (1994). Cytoarchitectonic anomalies in a genetically based disorder: Williams syndrome. *NeuroReport, 5,* 757–758.

Hickok, G., Neville, H., Mills, D., Jones, W., Rossen, M., & Bellugi, U. (1995). Electrophysiological and quantitative MR analysis of the cortical auditory system in Williams syndrome. *Cognitive Neuroscience Society Abstracts, 2,* 66.

Jernigan, T. L., & Bellugi, U. (1990). Anomalous brain morphology on magnetic resonance images in Williams syndrome and Down syndrome. *Archives of Neurology, 47,* 529–533.

Jernigan, T. L., & Bellugi, U. (1994). Neuroanatomical distinctions between Williams and Down syndromes. In S. Broman & J. Grafman (Eds.), *Atypical cognitive deficits in developmental disorders: Implications for brain function* (pp. 57–66). Hillsdale, NJ: Erlbaum.

Jernigan, T. L., Wang, P. P., & Bellugi, U. (1995). Neuromorphological characteristics of Williams syndrome. Special Issue, *Genetic Counseling, 6,* 145–146.

Jones, W., Bellugi, U., Lai, Z., Chiles, M., Reilly, J., Lincoln, A., & Adolphs, R. (chap. 2). Hypersociability: The social and affective phenotype of Williams Syndrome.

Jones, W., Lai, Z. L., & Bellugi, U. (February, 1999). Relations between cerebellar vermal areas and neuropsychological performance in Williams syndrome. *Journal of the International Neuropsychological Society, 5,* 152.

Korenberg, J., Chen, X.-N., Hirota, H., Lai, Z., Bellugi, U., Burian, D., Roe, B., & Matsoka, R. (chap. 6). Genome structure and cognitive map of Williams Syndrome.

Korenberg, J. R., Chen, X.-N., Lai, Z., Yimlamai, D., Bisighini, R., & Bellugi, U. (1997a). Williams syndrome: The search for the genetic origins of cognition. *American Journal Human Genetics, 61,* 103.

Korenberg, J. R., Chen, X.-N., Mitchell, S., & Sun, Z.-G. (1997b). The genomic organization of Williams syndrome. *International Behavioral Neuroscience Society Abstracts, 6,* 59.

Korenberg, J. R., Chen, X.-N., Mitchell, S., Sun, Z.-G., Hubert, R., Vataru, E. S., & Bellugi, U. (1996). The genomic organization of Williams syndrome. *American Society for Human Genetics Supplement, 59,* A304.

Korenberg, J. R., Hirota, H., Chen, X.-N., Lai, Z., Yimlamai, D., Matsuoka, R., & Bellugi, U. (1998). *The molecular genetic basis of Williams syndrome.* Presentation in symposium, Bridging cognition, brain and gene: Evidence from Williams syndrome. Abstract, Cognitive Neuroscience Society 1998 Annual Meeting Abstract Program, 11.

Lenhoff, H. M., Wang, P. P., Greenberg, F., & Bellugi, U. (1997). Williams syndrome and the brain. *Scientific American, 277,* 68–73.

Lowery, M., Morris, C., Ewart, A., Brothman, L., Zhu, X., Leonard, C., Carey, J., Keating, M., & Rothman, A. (1995). Strong correlations of elastin deletions, detected by FISH, with Williams syndrome: Evaluation of 235 patients. *American Journal of Human Genetics, 57,* 49–53.

Mills, D. L. (1998). *Electrophysiological markers for Williams syndrome.* Presentation in symposium, Bridging cognition, brain and gene: Evidence from Williams syndrome. Abstract, Cognitive Neuroscience Society 1998 Annual Meeting Abstract Program, 10.

Mills, D., Alvarez, T., St. George, M., Applebaum, L., Bellugi, U., & Neville, H. (chap. 3). Neurophysiological markers of face processing in Williams Syndrome.

Mills, D., Neville, H., Appelbaum, G., Prat, C., & Bellugi, U. (1997). Electrophysiological markers of Williams syndrome. *International Behavioral Neuroscience Society Abstracts, 6,* 59.

Neville, H., Mills, D., & Bellugi, U. (1995). Functional brain organization in Williams syndrome. Abstract, Special Issue, *Genetic Counseling, 6,* 141–142.

Osborne, L. R., Herbrick, J., Greavette, T., Heng, H. H. Q., Tsui, L.-C., Scherer, S. (1997a). PM52-related genes flank the rearrangement breakpoints associated with Williams syndrome and other diseases on human chromosome 7. *Genomics, 45,* 402–406.

Osborne, L. R., Sodar, S., Shi, X.-M., Pober, B., Costa, T., Scherer, S. W., & Tsui, L.-C. (1997b). Hemizygous deletion of the syntaxin 1A gene in individuals with Williams syndrome. *American Journal of Human Genetics, 61,* 449–452.

Perez-Jurado, L. A., Wang, Y. K., Peoples, R., Coloma, A., Cruces, J., & Francke, U. (1998). A duplicated gene in the breakpoint regions of the 7q11.23 Williams-Beuren syndrome deletion encodes the initiator binding protein TFII-I and BAP-135, a phosphorylation target of BTK. *Human Molecular Genetics, 7,* 325–334.

Reiss, A., Eliez, S., Schmitt, J. E., Strous, E., Lai, Z., Jones, W., & Bellugi, U. (chap. 4). Neuroanatomy of Williams Syndrome: A high-resolution MRI study.

Sawchenko, P., Dargusch, R., Arias, C., & Bellugi, U. (1997). Evidence for elastin expression in cerebellar Purkinje cells: Implications for Williams syndrome. *International Behavioral Neuroscience Society Abstracts, 6,* 59.

Wang, P. P., Doherty, S. D., Hesselink, J. R., & Bellugi, U. (1992). Callosal morphology concurs with neurobehavioral and neuropathological findings in two neurodevelopmental disorders. *Archives of Neurology, 49,* 407–411.

Wang, Y. K., Samos, C. H., Peoples, R., Perez-Jurado, L. A., Nusse, R., & Francke, U. (1997). A novel human homologue of the *Drosophila* frizzled wnt receptor gene binds wingless protein and is in the Williams syndrome deletion at 7q11.23. *Human Molecular Genetics, 6,* 465–472.

6 Genome Structure and Cognitive Map of Williams Syndrome

Julie R. Korenberg, Xiao-Ning Chen, Hamao Hirota, Zona Lai, Ursula Bellugi, Dennis Burian, Bruce Roe, and Rumiko Matsuoka

Williams syndrome (WMS) is a most compelling model of human cognition, of human genome organization, and of evolution. Due to a deletion in chromosome band 7q11.23, subjects have cardiovascular, connective tissue, and neurodevelopmental deficits. Given the striking peaks and valleys in neurocognition including deficits in visual-spatial and global processing, preserved language and face processing, hypersociability, and heightened affect, the goal of this work has been to identify the genes that are responsible, the cause of the deletion, and its origin in primate evolution. To do this, we have generated an integrated physical, genetic, and transcriptional map of the WMS and flanking regions using multicolor metaphase and interphase fluorescence in situ hybridization (FISH) of bacterial artificial chromosomes (BACs) and P1 artificial chromosomes (PACs), BAC end sequencing, PCR gene marker and microsatellite, large-scale sequencing, cDNA library, and database analyses. The results indicate the genomic organization of the WMS region as two nested duplicated regions flanking a largely single-copy region. There are at least two common deletion breakpoints, one in the centromeric and at least two in the telomeric repeated regions. Clones anchoring the unique to the repeated regions are defined along with three new pseudogene families. Primate studies indicate an evolutionary hot spot for chromosomal inversion in the WMS region. A cognitive phenotypic map of WMS is presented, which combines previous data with five further WMS subjects and three atypical WMS subjects with deletions; two larger (deleted for D7S489L) and one smaller, deleted for genes telomeric to *FZD9,* through *LIMK1,* but not *WSCR1* or telomeric. The results establish regions and consequent gene candidates for WMS features including mental retardation, hypersociability, and facial features. The approach provides the basis for defining pathways linking genetic underpinnings with the neuroanatomical, functional, and behavioral consequences that result in human cognition.

Introduction

Williams syndrome (WMS) is one of the most compelling models of human cognition. Given the emerging grasp of the human genome, study of subjects with WMS provides the opportunity to elucidate the pathways that lead from genes to behavior in the cognitive neurosciences. This understanding may ultimately help to shed light on our evolutionary origins and to elucidate a part of what makes us human.

WMS is a particularly powerful model, because it is characterized by specific deficits coupled with remarkably preserved abilities. It provides the opportunity to probe neurocognitive pathways in humans across different levels, including the cellular, physiological, anatomic, functional, and cognitive, with each of these ultimately related to the underlying changes in gene expression. Armed with this information, one can then begin to infer the interconnections and to understand the molecular basis of human behavior. In this report, the approach to defining the genetic, anatomic, and neurocognitive basis of WMS will be presented along with a physical map and the genomic structure of WMS region. These data will be used to generate a phenotypic map of WMS and to define subsets of genes responsible for a part of the facial features and mental retardation.

Physical Features and Neurocognition in WMS

WMS is a rare genetic disorder that occurs in about one in 25,000 births and is characterized by mental retardation, a hoarse voice, transient neonatal hypercalcemia, and a set of facial and physical features that includes cardiovascular defects, typically congenital supravalvular aortic stenosis (Table 6.1; Morris, Leonard, & Dilates, 1988; Morris, Loker, Ensing, & Stock, 1993). However, what is most striking about individuals with WMS is their unique cognitive profile. The power of WMS as a model for dis-

Table 6.1
Features of Williams Syndrome

Neurological	*Cardiovascular*
average IQ 55 (range 40–90)	supravalvular aortic stenosis
mild neurological dysfunction	peripheral pulmonary artery stenosis
tight heel cords	pulmonic valvular stenosis
poor coordination	ventricular/atrial septal defects
hyperacusis	
harsh, brassy or hoarse voice	*Musculoskeletal*
	joint limitations
Neurocognitive	kyphoscoliosis
friendly, loquacious personality	hallux valgus
musical ability	hypoplastic nails
relatively spared language development,	
enhanced vocabulary and social use of language	*Genitourinary*
compared to visual-spatial perception	nephrocalcinosis
	small, solitary, and/or pelvic kidneys
Facies	vesicouretal reflux
medial eyebrow flare	
short nasal palpebral fissures; epicanthal folds	*Endocrine*
flat nasal bridge	transient infantile hypercalcemia
stellate iris	
long philtrum	
prominent lips with open mouth	

Structure of the Region Deleted in Williams Syndrome

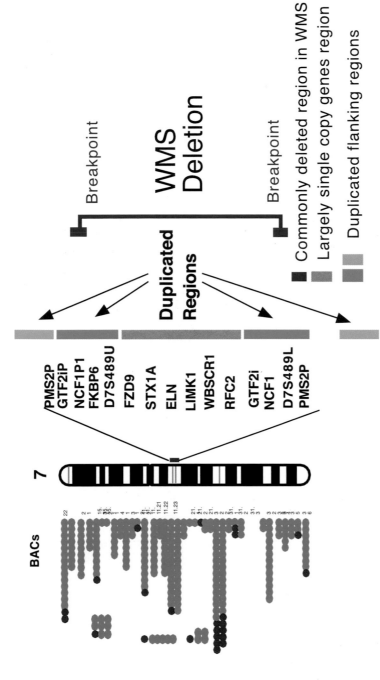

Plate 1 [Figure 6.1] The region of chromosome 7, band 7q11.23, that is commonly deleted in WMS is represented by the red box in the ideogram. This region is expanded at the right to illustrate its genomic organization, a region of largely single-copy genes flanked by a series of genomic duplications (as indicated by bars) containing genes (e.g., *GTF2i*), pseudogenes (e.g., *GTF2i*, *PMS2P*), and duplicate markers (e.g., *D7S489*). The regions used in the common breakpoints are indicated by red bars. The map positions of independent BACs used in part for this analysis are shown as green dots to the left of the ideogram.

Fluorescence In Situ Hybridization (FISH) of Williams Syndrome Chromosomes

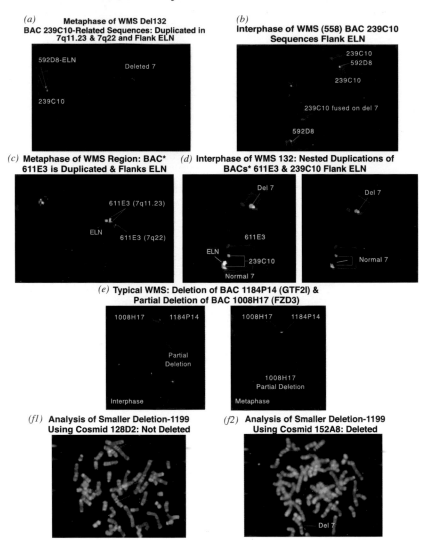

(a) Metaphase of WMS Del132
BAC 239C10-Related Sequences: Duplicated in
7q11.23 & 7q22 and Flank ELN

592D8-ELN
Deleted 7
239C10

(b) Interphase of WMS (558) BAC 239C10
Sequences Flank ELN

239C10
592D8
239C10
239C10 fused on del 7
592D8

(c) Metaphase of WMS Region: BAC*
611E3 is Duplicated & Flanks ELN

611E3 (7q11.23)
ELN
611E3 (7q22)

(d) Interphase of WMS 132: Nested Duplications of
BACs* 611E3 & 239C10 Flank ELN

Del 7
611E3
ELN
239C10
Normal 7

Del 7
Normal 7

(e) Typical WMS: Deletion of BAC 1184P14 (GTF2I) &
Partial Deletion of BAC 1008H17 (FZD3)

1008H17   1184P14
Partial
Deletion
Interphase

1008H17   1184P14
1008H17
Partial Deletion
Metaphase

(f1) Analysis of Smaller Deletion-1199
Using Cosmid 128D2: Not Deleted

(f2) Analysis of Smaller Deletion-1199
Using Cosmid 152A8: Deleted

Del 7

Plate 2 [Figure 6.2] BAC* indicates genomic sequences detected by and therefore presumed homologous to a given BAC. BAC* 239C10 (red) is duplicated within chromosome bands 7q11.23 as reflected by the large size of the signal on metaphase chromosomes (a), and signals are also seen in 7q22. As shown in the more extended DNA of interphase cells (b), BAC* 239C10 signals (red) flank the signals from BAC 592D8 (green) that carries the gene encoding elastin. (c) BAC* 611E3 (green) yields two clear signals within chromosome band 7q11.23, representing duplicated regions. The duplicated signals flank the single signal from BAC 592D8 (ELN) (red) as shown in metaphase chromosomes. (d) The duplicated signals from BAC 611E3 (red) surround those from BAC 239C10 (green) reflecting a nested duplication structure. Both signal sets flank the signal from BAC 592D8 (blue) as illustrated in these interphase cells. (e) BAC 1184P14 (green) carries the 5' region of the gene encoding GTF2I and is shown to be deleted in subjects with the common WMS deletion. BAC 1008H17 (red) carries the gene encoding FZD9 and generates a small signal, indicating partial deletion in subjects with the common WMS deletion (f1 and f2). Two cosmids detect different deletion patterns in WMS subject RM1199 with a smaller deletion. Cosmid 128D2 detects no deletion (f1), whereas cosmid 152A8 detects deletion (f2).

WMS Region Is a Hotspot in Primate Evolution

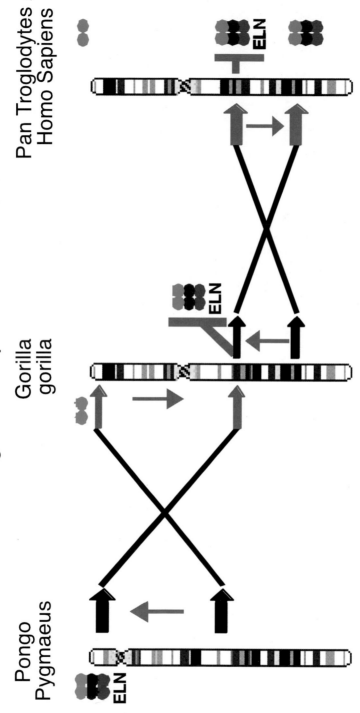

Plate 3 [Figure 6.4] The human chromosome 7 homologs from the orangutan (*Pongo*), gorilla (*Gorilla*), and chimpanzee (*Pan*) are illustrated. Horizontal arrows indicate the approximate chromosome band of the major inversions that have accompanied their speciation. Experiments using BACs from the closely flanking duplicated regions (BACs 239C10, 204, and 611E3) for FISH revealed duplicated sequences located at or close to all inversion breakpoints, illustrated by the colored dots. The gene for elastin (*ELN*) mapped to the subtelomeric band of Pongo, and was close to the initial inversion breakpoint in Pongo, and was close to the initial inversion breakpoint as well as all subsequent inversions cf chromosome 7 through primate evolution.

Model of Phenotype to Genotype Map of Williams Syndrome

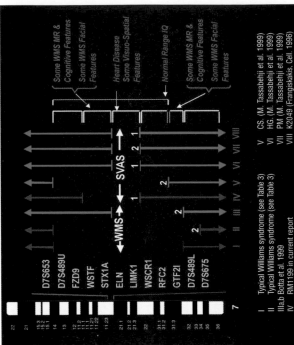

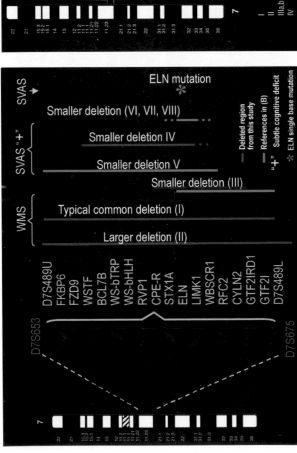

Plate 4 [Figure 6.5] Vertical lines on both figures indicate the regions deleted, and the number of subjects carrying the common WMS deletion associated with some of the typical facial features, mental retardation, and heart disease, the larger deletion associated with similar features, or the smaller deletions, that include subregions of Syntaxin1A through RFC2, associated with only the typical heart disease Supravalvar Aortic Stenosis (SVAS) and subtle cognitive deficits that fall within the normal range. Gene symbols are noted in the corresponding regions. Subject VIII has a subtle defect in visual spatial processing. * Indicates individuals with deletion or single base pair mutation of elastin, all associated only with SVAS and normal cognition. Small vertical brackets indicate deleted regions that differ among subjects, and therefore provide the potential to assign specific WMS features to single regions or genes. Some brackets indicate regions that, from the current data, are likely to contain a gene or genes that when deleted contribute in some measure to the WMS features denoted. The significance of these data is that deletion of *STXIA*, *ELN*, *LIMK1*, and *WSCR1*, and *RFC2* do not appear to be strongly associated with the characteristic facial or cognitive features seen in WMS, although they may contribute. In contrast, deletion of the region telomeric to *WSCR1* is associated with characteristic features of WMS cognition.

secting cognition lies in the distinct pattern of abilities and deficits. Individuals with WMS perform relatively well on tasks involving language and face processing, but show extreme difficulties on other aspects of spatial processing and auditory processing, particularly at the level of global organization (Bellugi, Wang, & Jernigan, 1994; Bellugi, Klima, & Wang, 1996; Bellugi, Lichtenberger, Mills, Galaburda, & Korenberg, 1999a; Bellugi, Mills, Jernigan, Hickok, & Galaburda, 1999b; Bellugi, Lichtenberger, Jones, Lai, & St. George, chap. 1). WMS is also associated with hyperacusis, an abnormal sensitivity to sound (Neville et al., 1994), although this is not linked to abnormalities in the peripheral auditory system. Finally, the prime characteristic of WMS individuals is a strong impulse toward social contact and affective expression (Jones et al., chap. 2; Bellugi & Wang, 1998; Bellugi, Losh, Reilly, & Anderson, 1998; Bellugi et al., 1999a; Reilly, Klima, & Bellugi, 1990) as well as a heightened sensitivity to music (Levitin & Bellugi, 1998).

The neurobiological profile of WMS is being revealed through the studies of brain function, structure, and cytoarchitechtonics. In these domains, specific event-related potentials (ERPs) have been defined as markers for aspects of face and language processing in WMS (Mills et al., chap. 3; Bellugi et al., 1999b; Neville, Mills, & Bellugi, 1994). Neuroanatomical studies employing MRI and histomorphometric approaches have revealed consistent morphological features of decreased overall cerebral cortical volume; spared limbic structures of the temporal lobe including the amygdala, hippocampus, and parahippocampal gyrus; larger neocerebellar vs. paleocerebellar lobules (Jernigan & Bellugi, 1994); and preservation in volume of Heschl's gyrus, an area in the primary auditory cortex (Reiss et al., chap. 4; Bellugi et al., 1999b; Galaburda, Wang, Bellugi, & Rossen, 1994; Galaburda & Bellugi, this volume). These features have been related to both the functional abnormalities and their possible embryological origins. Using the approach described, it is these neurocognitive and neurobiological features that will ultimately be combined with the genetic structure of WMS individuals to define the genes and pathways responsible.

Genetics of WMS

WMS is generally associated with a 1–2 Mb deletion of chromosome band 7q11.23 that includes the genes for elastin (Robinson et al., 1996; Gilbert-Dussardier et al., 1995; Nickerson, Greenberg, Keating, McCaskill, & Schaffer, 1995; Ewart et al., 1993), which is responsible for the congenital heart disease (Ewart, Jin, Atkinson, Morris, & Keating, 1994; Curran et al., 1993), LIM-kinase 1, which may contribute in part to the spatial deficit (Frangiskakis et al., 1996), and a growing number of other genes mapping in the region (illustrated in Figure 6.5). However, although WMS is clearly caused by the direct and downstream effects of genes located within the commonly deleted region, specific genes responsible for the major neurocognitive and physical features of WMS remain unknown. Gene candidates and transcripts mapping in the region include: *WSCR1–5* (Osborne et al., 1996); *RFC2,* the replication factor C subunit 2 (Peoples, Perez-Jurado, Wang, Kaplan, & Francke, 1996); *FZD9,* the human frizzled homolog of the *Drosophila wnt* receptor (Wang et al., 1997); *STX1A,* the syntaxin 1A gene (Osborne et al., 1997b); *GTF2I,* general transcription factor 2I (Perez-Jurado et al., 1998); WS-βTRP (WS-beta transducin repeats protein, ubiquitously expressed); *WS-bHLH* (a novel gene of the basic helix-loop-helix leucine zipper family of transcription factors that bind to E boxes, predominantly expressed in liver and kidney); *BCL7B,* a novel ubiquitously expressed gene (Meng et al., 1998); WSTF, WMS transcription factor (Lu, Meng, Morris, & Keating, 1998); FKBP6 (FK-506 binding protein, ubiquitously expressed); *CYLN2* (cytoplasmic linker-2 gene encoding the protein CLIP-115) (Hoogenraad et al., 1998); CPE-R (*Clostridium perfringens* enterotoxin receptor); and RVP1 (rat ventral prostate protein 1) (Paperna, Peoples, Wang, & Francke, 1998). In addition, the gene for NCF1 (neutrophil cytosolic factor 1) is located close to but is not deleted in WMS (Francke et al., 1990). It is not known which of these genes contributes to the phenotypic features of WMS. Using analyses of WMS subjects with atypical deletions, this report will illustrate the assignment of parts of the cognitive phenotype to the subsets of these genes.

Of importance for understanding both the cause and the phenotypic variability of WMS is the existence of genomic duplications that flank the largely unique region containing the genes described above. Both expressed genes and pseudogenes, as well as the breakpoints in the common WMS deletion, are thought to be located in these duplicated regions (Meng et al., 1998; Perez-Jurado et al., 1998; Osborne et al., 1997a; Korenberg et al., 1996; Robinson et al., 1996). However, the number of expressed genes in these duplicated regions and their contribution to the WMS phenotype is unknown. The current report will illustrate the structure of the flanking duplications and suggest a possible relationship to the WMS breakpoints.

In the current work, we will describe the construction of a working physical map of the WMS region including the flanking duplications. Combining data from fluorescence in situ hybridization (FISH), BAC end sequencing and large-scale sequence analyses, we will illustrate that the genomic organization of the WMS region includes two nested sets of duplications, the inner of which is involved in generating the common WMS deletion. A second gene for NCF1 will be shown to exist within the region deleted in some subjects with WMS. The genes for CPE-R and RVP1 have been assigned to single BACs. Three further gene fragments will be described and used to define the structure of the duplicated regions: *ATRA* (autoimmune thyroid antigen), a pseudogene for prohibitin that is located within an intron of the gene for GTF2i, and a novel gene that is duplicated but not deleted in WMS. Finally, using FISH and polymorphic marker analyses, we will describe the breakpoints in 78 individuals with WMS, two with larger deletions and one with a smaller deletion, and use this information to generate a phenotypic map of WMS, defining regions and genes likely to contribute independently to the mental retardation and to the facial features.

Data that describe progress in four areas will be presented below:

(a) The development of a physical map of the WMS region.

(b) Chromosomal breakpoints in WMS deletions.

(c) Evolution and human variation in the WMS region.

(d) The development of a phenotypic cognitive map of WMS.

Results

The Development of a Physical Map of the WMS Region: Chromosome Band 7q11.23

Using an approach that is independent of previous maps, we have generated an array of bacterial artificial chromosomes (BACs) (Korenberg et al., 1996, 1999a, Korenberg, Lai, & Bellugi, 1999b; http://www.csmc.edu/genetics/korenberg/korenberg.html) covering the human genome at random, each mapped at 2–6 Mb resolution by using FISH (Korenberg & Chen, 1995; Korenberg, Chen, Adams, & Venter, 1995). A subset of these was used to construct a BAC array with which to investigate the WMS region of chromosome 7 (see Figure 6.1) because yeast artificial chromosome (YAC) arrays of this region were highly rearranged and deleted (http://www.genet.sickkids.on.ca/chromosome7). Forty-five of the initial 233 BACs mapping to chromosome 7 were located on band 7q11.2, of which 30 generated single and 15 generated large or clearly double signals along each of the sister chromatids within band 7q11.23, suggesting a local duplication within this band (Korenberg et al., 1996). A subset of these duplicated BACs also generated signals in band 7q22, suggesting the existence of sequences in 7q22 that were homologous to those in 7q11.23, extending previous reports of multiple pseudogene family members located in these bands (Nicolaides et al., 1995). PCR analyses revealed that BAC 592D8 carried the gene for elastin. To further establish the genomic organization of the region with respect to the elastin deletion associated with WMS, a series of three- and four-color FISH experiments was conducted on normal and WMS chromosome preparations. These experiments employed pairs of duplicated BACs that were hybridized simultaneously with single-copy BACs previously known to map within band 7q11.23. The results illustrated in Figure 6.1 indicated that BACs containing elastin (592D8 and 1148G3), and two further randomly defined BACs (155B1 and 363B4),

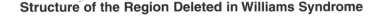

Structure of the Region Deleted in Williams Syndrome

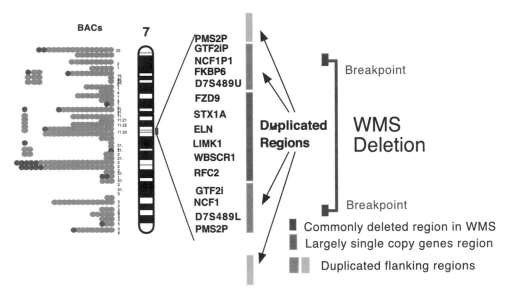

Figure 6.1
The region of chromosome 7, band 7q11.23, that is commonly deleted in WMS is represented by the red box in the ideogram. This region is expanded at the right to illustrate its genomic organization, a region of largely single-copy genes flanked by a series of genomic duplications (as indicated by bars) containing genes (e.g., *GTF2i*), pseudogenes (e.g., *GTF2i, PMS2P*), and duplicate markers (e.g., D7S489). The regions used in the common breakpoints are indicated by red bars. The map positions of independent BACs used in part for this analysis are shown as green dots to the left of the ideogram.

defined a single-copy region that was flanked by two nested duplicated regions. The inner duplicated region was defined by sequences related to BAC 239C10 and more closely flanked elastin (Figure 6.2a and b). The outer duplicated region was defined by signals generated by BAC 611E3 (Figure 6.2c), that flanked the signals generated by BAC 239C10. This is shown in Figure 6.2d in which four-color interphase FISH analysis reveals BAC 592D8 surrounded by duplicate signals from BAC 239C10 that are in turn, flanked by duplicate signals generated by BAC 611E3. The interphase analyses of WMS subjects' chromosomes shown in Figure 6.2a, b, and d, revealed that the signals from the inner duplicated region appeared to fuse on the deleted chromosome (2b), whereas the outer layer of signals was not affected (2d). This suggested that the sequences identified by BAC 239C10 were close to or included in a common breakpoint responsible for the WMS deletion and is further discussed below.

The resulting model of layered duplications flanking a largely single-copy genomic region containing elastin is shown in Figures 6.1 and 6.3. It was inferred that this

Fluorescence in Situ Hybridization (FISH) of Williams Syndrome Chromosomes

(a) **Metaphase of WMS Del132**
BAC 239C10-Related Sequences: Duplicated in
7q11.23 & 7q22 and Flank ELN

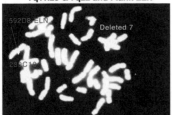

(b)
Interphase of WMS (558) BAC 239C10
Sequences Flank ELN

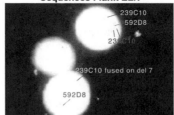

(c) **Metaphase of WMS Region: BAC***
611E3 is Duplicated & Flanks ELN

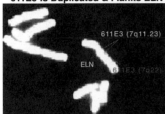

(d) **Interphase of WMS 132: Nested Duplications of**
BACs* 611E3 & 239C10 Flank ELN

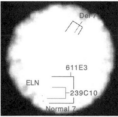 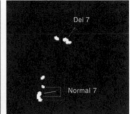

(e) **Typical WMS: Deletion of BAC 1184P14 (GTF2I) &**
Partial Deletion of BAC 1008H17 (FZD3)

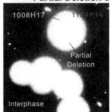 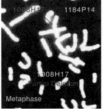

(f1) **Analysis of Smaller Deletion-1199**
Using Cosmid 128D2: Not Deleted

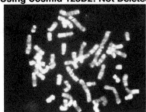

(f2) **Analysis of Smaller Deletion-1199**
Using Cosmid 152A8: Deleted

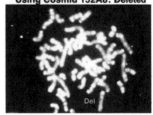

Figure 6.2

BAC* indicates genomic sequences detected by and therefore presumed homologous to a given BAC. BAC* 239C10 (red) is duplicated within chromosome bands 7q11.23 as reflected by the large size of the signal on metaphase chromosomes (a), and signals are also seen in 7q22. As shown in the more extended DNA of interphase cells (b), BAC* 239C10 signals (red) flank the signals from BAC 592D8 (green) that carries the gene encoding elastin. (c) BAC* 611E3 (green) yields two clear signals within chromosome band 7q11.23, representing duplicated regions. The duplicated signals flank the single signal from BAC 592D8 (ELN) (red) as shown in metaphase chromosomes. (d) The duplicated signals from BAC 611E3 (red) surround those from BAC 239C10 (green) reflecting a nested duplication structure. Both signal sets flank the signal from BAC 592D8 (blue) as illustrated in these interphase cells. (e) BAC 1184P14 (green) carries the 5′ region of the gene encoding GTF2I and is shown to be deleted in subjects with the common WMS deletion. BAC 1008H17 (red) carries the gene encoding FZD9 and generates a small signal, indicating partial deletion in subjects with the common WMS deletion. (f1 and f2) Two cosmids detect different deletion patterns in WMS subject RM1199 with a smaller deletion. Cosmid 128D2 detects no deletion (f1), whereas cosmid 152A8 detects deletion (f2).

A Physical and Transcript Map of the WMS Region

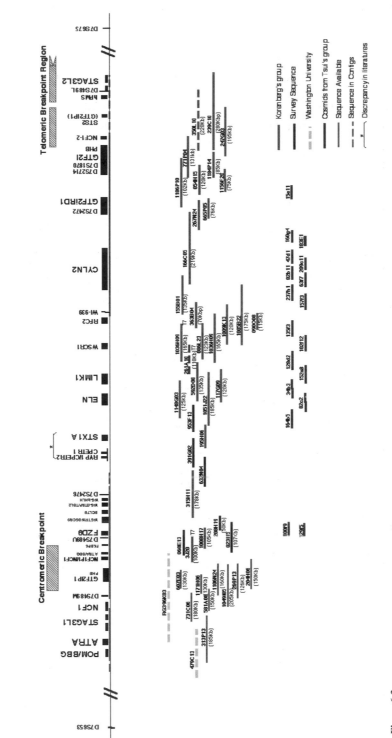

Figure 6.3

Genes and pseudogenes mapping in the WMS region are represented by black boxes (names reading vertically). BAC, PAC, and cosmid clones spanning this region are indicated below the genes and described in the Methods. The clones hybridized by using cDNA BAP135 are indicated by *, the clones hybridized by using cDNA PMS2 are indicated by +, and the clones of uncertain map position are indicated by 0. The relative locations of genes, microsatellite markers, and clones was confirmed by using PCR analysis. The location of BAC 611E3 is indicated by the patterned box and is not linked to the remaining contiguous clones. The open box for CYLN2 indicates unknown location of the 3' end.

duplicated structure was likely predisposed to the deletion responsible for WMS by meiotic mispairing.

STS and Southern Analyses Order the Duplicated Regions and Identify Clones that Anchor the Unique to the Repeated Regions at the Inner Borders of the Duplications   The model and organization of the two duplicated regions was further investigated by the analysis of BACs recognizing duplicated regions. This employed BAC to BAC Southern blots; sizing by pulsed field gel analyses; PCR (see Methods for table) and Southern analyses of ordered polymorphic and STS linked markers and the products of cDNA selection; sequencing and analysis of BAC ends; and analysis of expressed sequence tags (ESTs) developed from sequencing BAC 239C10. Details of STS analyses including end sequences will be presented elsewhere. BAC to BAC Southern blots employed the 45 BAC DNAs mapping in 7q11.2 digested with *Eco*RI probed with whole BAC DNAs (BAC to BAC Southerns). These revealed cohybridization of BACs in the duplicated regions that confirmed the BAC groupings (239C10 related, 611E3 related, and closer relatedness of 607E3 with 731C6), than of all other BACs carrying the marker D7S489M, including 581A8, 1106N4, and 1049I5. BAC to BAC Southerns also indicated the overlap of BACs 363B4 and 155B1 in the single-copy region, the overlap of single-copy BAC 697G1 with duplicated BACs 611 E3. PCR analyses with single-site polymorphic markers shown on the map D7S489L(A), D7S489U(B), D7S489M(C) (Perez-Jurado et al., 1998; Osborne et al., 1996, 1997a; Robinson et al., 1996), permitted the assignment of BACs from the duplicated regions to the centromeric or telomeric side of the single-copy region as illustrated (Figure 6.3), with 239C10 location later confirmed by continuity of DNA sequence from telomeric markers and large-scale sequence of BAC 350L10. As a way of determining the correct overlap in such highly related regions, the sequencing of BAC ends was used to exclude or to confirm overlap but, because of the extensive sequence duplication and conservation within the duplicated region, was rarely useful for definitive overlap. Given the high sequence homology determined from initial BAC end sequencing, the overlap of BACs without anchored markers was determined by best fit of all analyses. BACs that are highly duplicated and without anchoring polymorphic markers remain without definitive map assignment and are indicated in the map by diamonds. For example, although STS analyses for BACs 1171H6, 607E3, and 247G3 were compatible with both centromeric and telomeric locations, BAC to BAC Southerns suggested location as shown in Figure 6.3. In summary, from FISH, DNA sequence, and genomic Southern data, the duplications flanking the WMS region appeared to consist of multiple regions of highly homologous DNA sequences.

Anchor clones were defined in a manner that linked the single-copy region to the flanking centromeric and telomeric duplicated regions. These were 1008H17 (centromeric), that was initially identified at random and by PCR, was then found to carry both duplicated D7489U(B) and single-copy sequences of FZD9, both of which are deleted in the common WMS deletion (Wang et al., 1997). Therefore, it was clear that both single-copy and duplicated sequences were deleted in the common deletion. Moreover, this established the clone (1008H17) as carrying sequences that included the border of the single-copy and duplicated regions. FISH using this clone (1008H17 with FZD9) indicated that most individuals with WMS were partially deleted (Figure 6.2e). Further evidence supported this clone or the overlapping P1 artificial chromosome (PAC) 3J20 as containing the common breakpoint for the WMS deletion. This was suggested because PAC 3J20 carried both the commonly deleted marker D7489U and the nondeleted marker, *GTF2IP*, a pseudogene for the true gene, *GTF2I*, which is located at the telomeric end of the WMS common deletion (Perez-Jurado et al., 1998). Therefore, clones 1008H17 or 3J20 must contain the common centromeric breakpoint for WMS.

BAC clones anchoring the telomeric end of the single-copy region to the duplicated region, 1184P14 and 1156F20, were identified by screening for the unique marker D7S1870. These were found by BAC Southern analyses to carry a duplicated gene, initially called *BAP135* (data not shown), and then were confirmed to carry the 5′ STSs of the expressed form of the gene recently identified as *GTF2I* that is deleted in WMS (Perez-Jurado et al., 1998). This clone is deleted in all subjects with the common WMS deletion (Figure 6.2e), providing a reagent with which to define the telomeric end of the common WMS deletion.

Clone 611E3 May Anchor the Telomeric Duplicated Region to the Flanking Unique Region Located at the Border of Bands 7q11.23 and 7q21.1   The border between the telomeric duplicated region and the flanking single-copy region may be located close to or within BACs 611E3 or 697G1 since both carry the single-copy STS marker D7S2323, that is located telomeric to D7S489L, located in the telomeric duplication. BAC 697G1 is single copy (by FISH criteria) and maps by FISH to the border of bands 7q11.23-21. However, given the highly reduplicated nature of the entire region, the possibility remains that there are further duplicated regions flanking that defined by BAC611E3. Moreover, even the putatively single-copy STS, D7S2323, may itself be duplicated, and another copy of it located on the centromeric side of the WMS deleted region or in band 7q22. Nonetheless, these data suggest that there are regions in 7q11.23 that have been duplicated but are not involved in generating the WMS deletion.

Duplications Flanking the Elastin Region Contain Highly Conserved Gene Duplications and Processed Pseudogenes Originating from Many Chromosomes   Gene sequences for NCF1, ATRA, and prohibitin are duplicated in the centromeric and telomeric regions flanking the WMS deletion. To further investigate duplicated genes and to establish their potential relationship to the WMS deletion and phenotype, BAC 239C10 was partially sequenced and, along with BAC end sequences, was analyzed by database comparisons using BLAST searches (Altschul et al., 1997). Previously known genes located in the single-copy deleted region *(ELN, LIMK1, WSCR1, RFC2, STX1A, FZD9)*, in the putatively nondeleted *(NCF1* or neutrophil cytosolic factor 1), and in the duplicated regions *(PMS2)* were used to analyze all single and duplicated BACs by PCR, BAC Southern blots and sequence analyses of BAC 239C10. The gene for NCF1, previously mapped to 7q11.23 (Francke et al., 1990), but not thought deleted, was revealed to have at least three copies in the duplicated regions, two centromeric and one telomeric, by using a cDNA hybridized to BAC Southerns (data not shown). BAC 239C10 sequence analysis revealed a complete copy of the gene with a one-hundred-percent match to the published cDNA, and conservation of the appropriate intron/exon boundary sequences, located about 13 kb telomeric to the 3' end of *GTF2I* and transcribed centromere to telomere. However, comparison of the genomic sequence containing this *NCF1* gene, with the genomic sequence of NCF1 that had been previously determined (Gorlach et al., 1997), revealed numerous changes within the introns. Therefore, this new copy of the *NCF1* gene, located in BAC 239C10, was considered to be an *NCF1* gene duplication and possibly expressed. The previously described copy of *NCF1* was inferred to be likely located in the centromeric duplication, defined by the previous genomic sequence (Gorlach et al., 1997). Nonetheless, differences within introns or in more extended regions at intron/exon boundaries may alter the likelihood of expression. No further sequences matching *NCF1* were found in BAC 239C10 or in the overlapping BAC 350L11. In summary, as begun above, further analyses of the regions flanking the common WMS deletion indicate long stretches of conserved and highly homologous DNA.

Sequence analysis of BAC 239C10 also revealed further genes or fragments located within the duplicated regions. For example, a one-hundred-percent match to all but the 5' end of the gene *BAP135 (GTF2I)* was found within the centromeric 9 kb, along with matches to other exons located in an unlinked 34 kb contig. It was shown to be duplicated by Southerns in at least one further copy on the centromeric duplication. Recent work (Perez-Jurado et al., 1998) has confirmed the locations of this gene, now renamed *GTF2I,* and its centromeric pseudogene, along with the intron/exon structure. STSs from these cDNAs, conserved at close to one hundred percent for all but the unique 5' regions, were then used in the present analysis and are summarized in Figure 6.3. Further BAC 239C10 sequence analyses revealed the presence of a processed pseudogene for the prohibitin gene, containing numerous stop codons, and located at the centromeric end within intron 18 of *GTF2I* but transcribed in the opposite direction. The parent gene is located on chromosome 17q but PCR analyses revealed that sequences related to this gene were duplicated on all BACs containing *GTF2I*. This suggests that the insertion of the prohibitin pseudogene predated the formation of the duplications flanking the WMS region, and the degree of sequence drift separating the functional and the pseudogenes might be used as a molecular clock to estimate the time since and evolutionary origin of the duplicated regions. Finally, the marker D7S489L was also confirmed to exist on BAC 239C10, as were pseudogenes for PMS2. Members of the PMS2 family of pseudogenes were previously known to be located in bands 7q11.2, 7p22, 7p13, and 7q22 (Nicolaides et al., 1995). The number of pseudogenes determined by PCR may underestimate the copy number determined by hybridization because of gene rearrangements or sequence drift. Nonetheless, because of their distribution (Korenberg, unpublished) the *PMS2* pseudogene family may provide an even more ancient tag than prohibitin for sequences that are ultimately responsible for the duplications flanking WMS.

Further gene fragments mapping in the duplicated regions were determined by end sequencing. For example, BAC 581A8 end sequence matched a gene fragment for ATRA (autoimmune thyroid disease-related antigen; M28639, Hirayu, Seto, Magnusson, Filetti, & Rapoport, 1987). Southern analyses revealed duplication as shown in Figure 6.2. Screening a brain cDNA library for the complete cDNA revealed an expressed pseudogene containing ATRA fused to a fragment from a novel gene isolated from a brain library (*BBG* in Figure 6.3) (Ishikawa et al., 1998) with both fragments located in multiple copies in the duplicated region. Further details will be reported elsewhere.

In order to determine the degree of homology and structure of the duplicated regions, Southern analyses were followed with sequencing of PCR fragments templated on BACs in the duplicated regions because, in most cases, identical fragment sizes were obtained from the Southern analyses. However, sequence analyses revealed a ninety-seven- to one-hundred-percent homology of sequences from BACs located on the two sides of the duplicated regions. The exceedingly high homology of some sequences flanking the WMS deleted region suggested either recent origin or a mechanism that selectively maintained homology; in either case, the high homology provides challenges to the genomic analysis and may predispose to mispairing at meiosis, thereby increasing genetic variability in this region.

Genes in the Single-Copy Region   To cover the single-copy region, PCR fragments from BAC end sequences (155B1, 363B4, 1184G3, 1008H17), mapped markers (D7S1870), and cDNA sequences (LIMK1, elastin) were used to screen the BAC library (Research Genetics, Huntsville, AL), followed by confirmation of overlap by

PCR. The map of the single-copy region was further confirmed by PCR of genes and markers indicated on the map and was linked to other ordered clone sets (Meng et al., 1998a; Meng, Lu, Morris, & Keating, 1998b; Paperna et al., 1998; Osborne et al., 1997a, 1997b) by PCR and Southern analyses. The genes for CPE-R (*Clostridium perfringens* enterotoxin receptor) and RVP-1 (rat ventral prostate 1 protein), both recently mapped to the region between STX1A and FZD9 (Paperna et al., 1998), were mapped to PAC 391G2 by PCR. All putatively single-copy genes were evaluated for possible duplication by PCR and hybridization to BACs from the duplicated regions. Further cosmids and PACs obtained as indicated from other groups, were confirmed by PCR and Southerns to overlap as shown on the map in Figure 6.3.

The conclusion from these experiments was that the WMS region of band 7q11.2 was composed of a largely single-copy region of about 1.5 Mb containing at least 19 known genes. This region is flanked by duplications containing highly conserved processed and unprocessed pseudogenes, some of which are transcribed and many with homologies of ninety-nine percent. The next critical questions were to determine which of the single copy and which of the duplicated genes and pseudogenes were deleted in subjects with WMS and of these, which were important for determining the phenotype. To do this, the map reagents and information were then used to determine the regions and genes deleted in subjects diagnosed with WMS.

Chromosomal Breakpoints in WMS Deletions

The Inner Duplication Is Involved in the WMS Common Deletion   Next, the BAC map reagents were used to determine the regions deleted in WMS subjects, to estimate the size of the deletion, and to define closely flanking markers. To do this, each of the 40 initial BACs randomly mapping in 7q11.2 was tested singly on metaphase and interphase chromosomes from six WMS subjects and evaluated with respect to the deleted chromosome using simultaneous hybridization of a control BAC located in band 7q22. The results illustrated in Figure 6.2 for BAC 239C10, clearly showed that the signals from BACs 239C10 and 731C6 that flanked elastin, were now joined in a single, smaller signal on the chromosome carrying the deletion whereas the duplicated signals from BAC 611E3, that flanked the 239C10 duplicated region now moved closer on the deleted chromosome but were not joined, as shown in Figure 6.2. BAC 731C6 generated smaller, more defined signals on interphase analyses. A third pattern was seen by BAC 204H6, which generated duplicated signals that were more diffuse and more closely surrounding the single-copy region (data not shown). These results suggested that the deletion breakpoints were located within or very close to the sequences recognized by BAC 239C10 and that part of the duplicated region was itself deleted.

WMS Chromosomes Delete Parts of the Clones that Anchor the Unique and Duplicated Regions   To determine the regions commonly deleted in WMS, 74 subjects with clinically diagnosed WMS were tested as above. Chromosome preparations from subjects and 20 parents were analyzed by simultaneous FISH for BACs carrying elastin (592D8, 1051J22, 1148G3), the telomeric anchor clone that contained the gene for GTF2I, 1184P14; 239C10, and for 28 cases, the centromeric anchor BAC, 1008H17 (carrying the gene *FZD9*). The results summarized in Table 6.2, indicate that 73 of 74 subjects, but none of the parents (data not shown), were deleted for all single-copy BACs including the distal anchor marker. The common WMS deletion and the genes consequently deleted are shown in Figure 6.5. All save one were also partially deleted for the centromeric flanking marker 1008H17 and for BACs marking the flanking duplications (e.g., 239C10). The single case without a deletion was felt, on review, not to be typical, but, nonetheless, requires further study. This suggested that anchor BAC 1008H17 contained the centromeric breakpoint and that BAC 239C10 contained the telomeric breakpoint. Interphase analyses indicated that PAC 3J20 mapped on top of 1008H17, supporting it as the anchor and proximal breakpoint marker. The conclusion from this analysis was that the breakpoints of the common WMS deletion were not grossly variable but were rather clustered in a small region close to the centromeric and telomeric borders between the unique and repeated regions. This suggested that most subjects with WMS were deleted for roughly the same regions, and, therefore, variability in neurocognitive phenotype was not likely determined by large differences in gene content.

Table 6.2
Analysis of Deletion in WMS Subjects Using FISH with BAC Clones and Microsatellites of Parents and Proband

Markers	No. Deleted/No. Subjects Tested	No. Deleted/No. Informative*, $n = 112$	Deleted (%)
FISH with BACs			
FZD3 (B1008H17)	27/28		96.4
ELN + LIMK1(B592D8)	73/74		98.6
RFC2 (B155B1)	8/8		100
GTFWI (B1184P14)	58/59		98.3
Microsatellites			
D7S653	34	25/25	100
D7S489U	36	9/9	100
D7S1870	39	26/26	100
D7S489L	34	2/11	18.2
D7S849	39	2/16	12.5
D7S675	38	0/25	0

*from ABI Analysis

It remained possible that genes at or near the breakpoints or within the duplicated regions, could contribute disproportionately to the classical WMS features. This spurred the search for rare subjects with smaller deletions.

WMS Subjects with Atypical Deletions To further determine the extent of the deletions, particularly within the duplicated regions, microsatellite markers D7S489M, D7S489U, D7S1870, D7S489L, D7S849 (all except D7S489M, previously reported as deleted with variable frequencies), and the flanking markers, D7S675 and D7S653, were analyzed in parents and probands from 40 families. This revealed that 11 of the 40 probands were informative for D7S489L, and two of these 11 were deleted. All of the 26 informative probands were deleted for D7S1870, but not for the flanking markers (D7S675 and D7S653). A subset of phenotypic features for the two subjects with the atypical larger deletions are shown in Table 6.3 and the molecular data are shown in Figure 6.5. Both revealed typical WMS features. In addition, a further subject (data not shown), also carried a larger deletion and exhibited hyperlexia (ability to phonologically decode written words without necessarily comprehending them). Full neurocognitive analyses are reported elsewhere (Korenberg et al., 1999a). In summary, the phenotypic features of WMS subjects with the common deletion or with the larger deletion are similar but may possess subtle neurocognitive differences that merit further study.

WMS subjects with smaller deletions were first identified by screening using FISH with the anchor BAC clones, 1184P14 and 1008H17, and BAC 592D8 (elastin) as reported elsewhere for Italian subjects, (Botta et al., 1999) and in a study of Japanese subjects. The clinical features of these along with those in the literature are shown in Table 6.3. One subject, RM1199, was found to be deleted for BAC 592D8 but for neither of the anchoring BACs. This 8-year-old girl had SVAS, a broad nasal tip, a slightly thick lower lip, dental anomalies, mild mental retardation, with a normal birth history. No further clinical information was available and photographs were not permitted. Further analyses employed the reagents from the map (Figure 6.3) for FISH (BACs 239C10, 315H11, 1148G3, 363B4, 155B1, PACs P632N4, 391G2, 195h6, 953F13, 261A10, 267N24, cosmids 129F5, 82C2, 152a8, 128d2, 15e3, 183e1, 209c11, and 82b11), and quantitative Southern blot dosage analysis (data not shown) for the gene *FZD9*. The results (shown in Figure 6.2f and later in Figure 6.5) revealed the deletion of all contiguous clones from B632N$_4$ through cos152a8 but the presence of the overlapping anchor clones, B1008H17 and 129f5, indicating no apparent deletion of *FZD9* (confirmed by Southern analysis using gene-specific hybridization), but deletion for the remainder of the region including the genes telomeric to *FZD9*, viz., *STX1A*, *CPE-R*, *RVP1*, and *ELN*, and likely also for the genes, carried on the deleted BAC B632N$_4$. The

Table 6.3
Phenotypes of Atypical WMS Subjects

SUBJECT PHENOTYPE GROUP	I	II	IIIa	IIIb	IV	V	VI	VII
Age at Exam (Yr)	11Y	13.3Y	6Y	2Y				
SEX								
Male	●			●			●	●
Female		●	●		●	●		
GROWTH								
Weight %	95	7	97	3				
Height %	25	10	50	10				
Head Circ. %	10		25	10				
Birth weight low				+				
PHYSICAL FEATURES								
Face	+	+	+	+		−	−	−
Bulbous nasal tip/ short	+/+	−/+	+/+	+	+	−	−	−
Lower lip thick	+	+	+	+/+	+			
Malar flat	−	+	+	+		−	−	−
Periorbital Fullness	−	+	+	+		−	−	−
Stellate Iris	−	+	+			−	−	−
Epicanthal Folds	+	+	+			−	−	−
Dental Anomalies					+			
Hoarse Voice	+	+						
Heart								
SVAS	−	+	+		+	+	+	+
PA Stenosis				+				
Renal Anomalies								
Hernia	−	+				−	−	−
BONY MALFORMATIONS								
Sloping Shoulders	+	+				−	−	−
Long Trunk	−	+				−	−	−
NEUROLOGICAL								
Abnormal Gait	+	+						
COGNITIVE								
Retardation								
Milestones Retarded	+	+	+(mild)	+	+(mild)			
IQ				68		normal	normal	normal
Cognitive profile						−	−	−
BEHAVIOR								
Hypersocial	+	+/−	+					

Note: For deletion size, see Figure 5a,b.

telomeric breakpoint revealed deletion of clones through *LIMK1* but not for *WSCR1* or for sequences further telomeric. In summary, the analysis of WMS subject RM1199 revealed an atypical smaller deletion: Neither *FZD9* nor *GTF2I* were deleted, but the genes located telomeric to *FZD9* through *WBSCR1* were deleted.

The molecular data and subsets of the clinical and cognitive information from the subjects was then combined with data from the larger deletions described above, from other reports of individuals with SVAS and other features accompanied by deletion (Botta et al., 1999; Tassabehji et al., 1997, 1999; Frangiskakis et al., 1996; Olson et al., 1995) or single-base mutation of elastin (Li et al., 1997), and was used to generate a cognitive map as shown in Figure 6.5. This revealed regions likely to contain genes, which are in part responsible for the mental retardation and facial features, and, possibly, for a part of the hypersociability seen in WMS.

Evolution and Human Variation in the WMS Region

The duplicated region surrounding the WMS deletion can be traced through the evolution of primate chromosomes. This was investigated to better understand the origin of the duplicated regions and because of the possibility that changes in gene content and expression in the WMS region could be in part responsible for changes accompanying speciation in primates as well as for variation in human cognition. To do this, the chromosomal locations of BAC probes for the duplicated regions (239C10 and 611E3) and for the single-copy region (elastin, 592D8) were evaluated in the orangutan *(Pongo pygmaeus)*, the gorilla *(Gorilla gorilla)*, and the chimpanzee *(Pan troglodytes)*. There have been two inversions in the higher primate homologues of human chromosome 7. The results, summarized in Figure 6.4, revealed that the region of 7q11.2 deleted in WMS has been involved in both of these evolutionary breakage and inversion events. The probes for both the duplicated and single-copy regions generated signals in the chromosome bands involved in the region of the inversions occurring between the orangutan and gorilla, and then again between the gorilla and the chimpanzee. It is of interest that the WMS region represented by BAC 239C10 was already partially duplicated in the orangutan, and appears to increase in signal with each inversion event, transferring part to the new site and leaving part of the duplicated region at the previous site, suggesting partial duplications associated with the inversions. The chimpanzee chromosome appears grossly similar in hybridization pattern to the human using the current probes but may vary for regions not yet tested. For all species changes, only the molecular analysis will allow an accurate understanding of the subtle rearrangements and potential duplications of these regions. Nonetheless, although such inversion and duplication is uncommon, it characterizes speciation during primate evolution. Therefore, we must ask to what extent these regions have contributed to primate speciation.

WMS Region Is a Hotspot in Primate Evolution

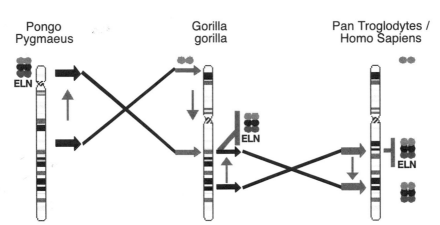

Figure 6.4
The human chromosome 7 homologs from the orangutan (*Pongo*), gorilla (*Gorilla*), and chimpanzee (*Pan*) are illustrated. Horizontal arrows indicate the approximate chromosome band of the major inversions that have accompanied their speciation. Experiments using BACs from the closely flanking duplicated regions (BACs 239C10, 204, and 611E3) for FISH revealed duplicated sequences located at or close to all inversion break-points, illustrated by the colored dots. The gene for elastin (*ELN*) mapped to the subtelomeric band of Pongo, and was close to the initial inversion breakpoint as well as all subsequent inversions of chromosome 7 through primate evolution.

Moreover, we must also ask whether humans are variable for these regions and for the expression of the genes within them, and to what extent might the normal variation of behavior in the cognitive domains we are looking at be determined by variation in these regions.

Discussion

The physical map of the WMS region presented in this report reveals that the commonly deleted region is flanked by nested duplicated regions that are linked to the STS maps (see Figure 6.3). The inner duplicated region corresponds to the previously noted duplications that included PMS2, D7S489, and GTF2I (Perez-Jurado et al., 1998; Osborne et al., 1996). The current report extends the understanding of this region and suggests that the outer duplicated region appears asymmetrically located with respect to the gene for elastin. Moreover, the current analysis that is summarized in Figure 6.3 reveals that some subsections of the region are oriented in part in parallel and others are not. Further, the duplications themselves appear to be scrambled, somewhat reminiscent of the duplications found in chromosome band 5q13, in which deletion is responsible for SMA1 (Campbell, Potter, Ignatius, Dubowitz, & Davies, 1997). Moreover, some duplicated pseudogenes (*ATRA, BBG,* prohibitin) may also be located in band 7q22 (data not shown). All of this suggests that the formation of these regions included numerous events that occurred over an extended time period during primate or earlier evolution. Moreover, until the structure is supported by sequence data, it is still possible that the unit defined by D7489M is located in or duplicated in the telomeric duplication, and given the apparent multiple nature of the D7S489M signals, it is possible that there are further copies, and that the entire region is polymorphic in the human population. If D7S489M is duplicated, and at least one copy lies outside the deleted region, this would call into question its use in defining the usual WMS breakpoint. Finally, the genomic duplication of *NCF1* found in BAC 239C10 is of interest because the exon sequences are ninety-nine percent homologous to the putative functional copy located in the centromeric duplication but the intronic regions vary, being only ninety-seven percent homologous. This suggests that the telomeric duplication represented by BAC 239C10 is of recent origin, likely after the chimpanzee, or that the homology is maintained by some other mechanism, possibly gene conversion. Further, although this suggests that the gene for NCF1 was expressed for some time after duplication and may still be expressed by both the present telomeric and previously reported presumptively centromeric copies, this is made less likely by the observation of an autosomal recessive form of CGD (chronic granulomatous disease) that is caused by deletion of a GT in NCF1. The autosomal recessive inheritance implies that both parental copies, and, by inference, both centromeric and telomeric copies, would have to be mutated. Further analyses may yield differences in expressive potential due to promoter or intron/exon junction sequences.

Deletion Breakpoints in WMS: One Centromeric and at Least Two Telomeric

The definition of marker D7S849 as telomeric to D7S489L and possibly deleted in at least two individuals suggests the existence of a second telomeric breakpoint as indicated on the map in Figure 6.3. Although both the centromeric break and the first telomeric break appear to be common to most WMS deletions, by the current report as well as by previous analyses (Perez-Jurado et al., 1998; Robinson et al., 1996), further work is necessary to determine if the second break is also clustered. The second breakpoint may be located close to the outer ring of duplicated regions defined by BAC 611E3. It is of interest that we have placed a third *NCF1* copy close to the *GTF2I* pseudogene in the centromeric break and that these same genes appear to characterize the telomeric break, suggesting that sequences at or beyond the GTFZI 3′ and the 5′ end of *NCF1,* may be involved in the deletion as suggested (Perez-Jurado et al., 1998). It is important to note that the cause of the deletion may include a number of factors including the high frequency of Alu elements in the region and the high degree of sequence conservation in the duplicated regions. However, the limited localization of the breakpoints augers that particular sequences or chromatin structures may be major contributors. Candidate sequences could include any number of elements associated with genome instability (e.g., mariner elements, L1, HERV, THE1, etc.), although none of these have been demonstrated as causative. Finally, it is of interest that BAC 611E3 may be located close to the 7q11.23-q21 border which delineates points at which stable replication forks must exist during DNA mitotic synthesis in that band q21 replicates late and band q11.23 earlier during the DNA synthetic period. The DNA structures that underlie the regions of band borders may themselves be unstable and may contribute to the tendency to delete.

We have, therefore, proposed that the repeat sequences illustrated by the BAC analyses are either responsible for or are caused by the same instabilities that lead to the deletion in WMS (Korenberg et al., 1997a, 1997b). In any event, it is likely that the meiotic mispairing of subsets of these sequence families combined with crossing-over (Robinson et al., 1996) results in a series of different chromosomal aberrations of the deletion/duplication types. Although these have not yet been described for the WMS region, similar duplicated structures on other chromosomes are also associated with deletions and rearrangements causing neurologic disease (Lupski, 1998). One fascinating aspect of this finding is the potential to define repeat sequence structures, and, therefore, other breakpoints and deletions that may be characteristic of particular phenotypes, adding another dimension to our understanding of genome organization and cognition.

Genes Responsible for Neurocognition, Neuroanatomy, and Behavior in WMS   The ultimate goal of this work was to understand the pathways that bridge genes and behavior by elucidating the genes deleted in different individuals with WMS, and by linking across levels, the information on gene expression, neuroanatomy, physiology, and neurocognition. To do this, we have presented the analysis of 74 subjects with clinically diagnosed WMS, which, together with other studies, has begun to show promise. The initial prospects for linking genotype and phenotype in WMS, with the traditional genetic approach, were grim since most all cases appeared to be deleted for the same region and the same genes (Perez-Jurado et al., 1998). Ideally, one would like to have seen some variability in the deletions and to link this with variations in cognitive behavior. Slowly, we are beginning to build up a database of these individuals who are partially deleted and show partial features of WMS. It is by combining the data from these subjects with other individuals carrying atypical deletions, that we have now begun to assign neurocognitive features of WMS to different regions with known genes.

The Development of a Phenotypic Cognitive Map of WMS

The result of combining the current molecular and cognitive data with the literature results in a suggestion of both the regions and the genes within that are ultimately involved in generating the phenotypic features of WMS. The current phenotypic map of WMS is shown in Figure 6.5a and b.

The map was constructed by using the clinical data shown in Table 6.3 with the following rationale. In WMS, there is ample room for justifiable speculation as to which genes should be responsible for the cognitive features of WMS. The gene for LIMK1 has been implicated (Frangiskakis et al., 1996) but not substantiated (Tassabehji et al., 1999) as a cause of the visual-spatial features of WMS, and the genes for STX1A and FZD9 have been implicated simply by their brain-specific gene expression in the developing (FZD9) or adult (STX1A) central nervous system. However, regardless of the theoretical attraction of these molecules as mediators of cognitive processes and their embryological substrata, it is important to test their significance in causing the phenotypes at hand when they are underexpressed by fifty percent as is likely in the WMS brain. When this is done, as illustrated in Figure 6.5, we see that deletion of these genes is not associated with the significant effects on overall cognition that are characteristic of WMS. Therefore, we must now ask not only which genes are likely to affect cognition, but simultaneously, which regions and their genes have been demonstrated in humans to be associated with changes in cognition when deleted. First, it is now clear that deletion of elastin is responsible for the cardiovascular defects of WMS, based on the effects of both small deletions and point mutations of elastin. It is also strongly suggested that none of the other physical features is largely due to deletion of elastin. This is based on the lack of these features (e.g., facies, hoarse voice) in individuals with elastin single-base mutations (Li et al., 1997). Second, although a part of the visual-spatial deficit may be due to deletion of LIMK1 (Frangiskakis et al., 1996), this is unlikely to be the major gene responsible as the observation is not supported by three further cases that delete this gene as well as others (Tassabehji et al., 1999; Figure 6.5). The strength of this inference is emphasized by one of the cases being an engineering student. Third, from case RM1199 reported here, who is deleted for the region from WSTF through WSCR1, and the case CS (Tassabehji et al., 1999), who carries a deletion of the region from FZD9 through RFC2, it appears unlikely that the genes in this region can be largely responsible for the characteristic WMS mental retardation, sociability, visual-spatial or memory deficits, language preservation, or facial features. This is because both of these individuals have heart disease with essentially normal range or mildly impaired cognitive and physical features. There-

Model for Phenotype to Genotype Map of Williams Syndrome

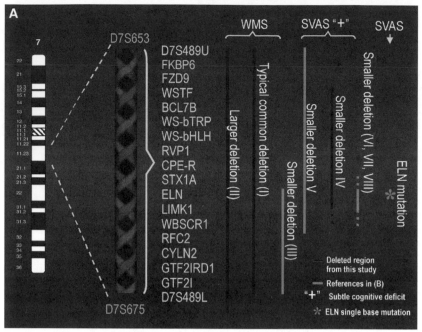

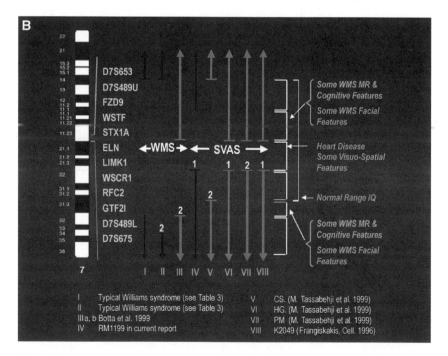

Figure 6.5
Vertical lines on both figures indicate the regions deleted, and the number of subjects carrying the common WMS deletion associated with some of the typical facial features, mental retardation, and heart disease, the larger deletion associated with similar features, or the smaller deletions, that include subregions of Syntaxin1A

fore, it is likely that the genes responsible for a major part of the mental retardation and other features are located in the region telomeric to *RFC2* through *GTF2I* at the telomeric border of the deletion. Nonetheless, the mild cognitive deficits seen in RM1199 and in one of the two subjects deleted for elastin and LIMK1 (Tassabehji et al., 1999) suggest that decreased expression of genes in the region from WSTF through LIMK1 are associated with subtle defects in cognition. The contribution of genes in the telomeric region to the facial features and mental retardation is supported by the classical facial features seen in individuals with deletions of *STX1A* through *GTF2I* (Botta et al., 1999). Finally, it is important to note that, similar to subjects with the common full WMS deletion, the cognitive deficits in individuals with small deletions are variable and understanding the range of consequences of single deleted genes requires study of further individuals.

This exciting initial map of cognition is important in setting out the approach for defining the other domains of cognitive function and neuroanatomic structure as described above. Moreover, it emphasizes that, with a small number of subjects, however rare, significant understanding can be gained. From the map it is appreciated that, even with the small number of subjects currently reported, seven different regions could be defined for cognitive phenotypes that were delineated clearly. It is the development of sensitive measures and their study in these and other rare individuals that will ultimately provide clues to the critical steps in the pathways of human cognition.

Caveats to the WMS Cognitive Map   It is important to note that the variable expression of genes that are not deleted may also be affected and contribute to phenotype. These may include the effects of transcribed but not translated pseudogenes including those for GTF2I. Further sources of phenotypic variability include interactions of genes in the deleted region with others mapping both in and outside of the WMS region as well as possible regional disturbances of replication and transcription due to deletion and rearrangement. Such larger rearrangements that do not result in deletion may yet be a cause of the WMS phenotype by such a mechanism. Some rearrangements may lead to the decreased expression of nondeleted genes, and to the incorrect association of genes

through RFC2, associated with only the typical heart disease Supravalvar Aortic Stenosis (SVAS) and subtle cognitive deficits that fall within the normal range. Gene symbols are noted in the corresponding regions. Subject VIII has a subtle defect in visual-spatial processing. * Indicates individuals with deletion or single base pair mutation of elastin, all associated only with SVAS and normal cognition. Small vertical brackets indicate deleted regions that differ among subjects, and therefore provide the potential to assign specific WMS features to single regions or genes. Some brackets indicate regions that, from the current data, are likely to contain a gene or genes that when deleted contribute in some measure to the WMS features denoted. The significance of these data is that deletion of *STX1A, ELN, LIMK1, WSCR1,* and *RFC2* do not appear to be strongly associated with the characteristic facial or cognitive features seen in WMS, although they may contribute. In contrast, deletion of the region telomeric to *WSCR1* is associated with characteristic features of WMS cognition.

with cognitive function. Ideally, gene expression in the brain both during fetal and adult life must be understood to assess this. However, the present map is a good beginning.

Other potential sources of genetic effects on cognition include imprinting, or the phenomenon by which the expression of a gene is differentially modified by passing through the maternal or the paternal germline. For WMS, this has been suggested for growth and head circumference (Pankau, Partsch, Neblung, Gosch, & Wessel, 1994; Francke, Yang-Feng, Brissenden, & Ulrich, 1986) and was recently investigated for a subset of the neurocognitive phenotypes (Korenberg et al., 1999). So far, it appears the parent of origin of the deletion is not related to the neurocognitive performance on any of the measures so far tested. These include overall intellectual ability, receptive and productive language, visual-spatial measures (with and without motor), and facial identification. However, other cognitive variables that have not yet been tested may be affected by the parent of origin. These may include memory (both verbal and visual, immediate, and long-term), conservation ability, frontal executive functions, friendliness and social behavior, and emotion perception. Although preliminary results indicated no significant difference, larger numbers of subjects and the development of more sensitive and specific measures may be required to elucidate more subtle effects of genetic imprinting on gene expression in WMS.

In summary, the data from studies of rare WMS subjects with atypical deletions are the most informative in identifying gene candidates for human cognitive features. Evidence suggests that mental retardation may be largely determined by the centromeric and telomeric regions and facial features determined at least in part determined by the telomeric region defined above. The next essential step is to parse the phenotype; to perform detailed cognitive, neuroanatomic, and physical studies of these individuals; and to devise and apply sensitive tests of musicality and sociability that probe the limits of these processes and that are informative across variation in intellectual function as seen in WMS. The multidimensional data from well-studied individuals with atypical deletions can thus be used to elucidate the many levels requiring intersection in the neurosciences; the role of neuroanatomic structures in cognition and behavior; and the role of gene expression in determining structure, cognition, and possibly disease.

Methods

Clinical Subjects, DNA Isolation, and Chromosome Preparation

Seventy-four WMS subjects used for this study were evaluated by the Laboratory for Cognitive Neuroscience at The Salk Institute for Biological Studies, La Jolla, CA. The procedures and consent forms were approved by The Salk Institute Institutional Review Board (IRB). DNAs were isolated either directly from peripheral blood or from lymphoblastoid cell lines using the Puregene DNA isolation Kit (Gentra, Minneapolis, MN) according to the manufacturer's instruction.

Chromosome preparations were generated by a standard technique from peripheral blood samples (Korenberg & Chen, 1995) for both humans and other primates. Primate bloods were obtained from the Yerkes Laboratory Yerkes Primate Research Institute/ Emory University.

BAC to BAC Southerns

The BAC DNA preparations and the size of each clone were performed according to the procedure described by Hubert et al., (1997). Briefly, BAC DNAs were isolated using miniprep or midiprep kits (Qiagen) with modifications. *Not*I digests excised the insert and provided a convenient means of determining the sizes of clones. Southern blots of *Not*I and *Eco*RI double-digests of miniprep or midiprep DNA were used to show overlaps between clones. To prepare probes from BACs, 50–100 ng of DNAs were labeled using random priming (Boehringer Manheim). The hybridization and wash conditions were as described previously (Korenberg et al., 1995).

FISH and Chromosomal Analysis

The BAC clones were confirmed and mapped to chromosome 7q by using multicolor FISH as described previously (Korenberg et al., 1995). One microgram of miniprep BAC DNA was either indirectly labeled with biotin-14-dUTP or digoxigenin-11-dUTP or directly labeled with Cy5-dUTP, Arcour-dUTP using nicktranslation kits (GIBCO BRL; Amersham). FITC-avidin (Vector Lab) and Rhodamine-antidigoxigenin (Boehringer Manheim) were used for the detection of biotinylated and digoxigenin labeled probes, respectively. The directly labeled probes were viewed immediately after the counterstaining with chromomycin A3 and distamycin A, which generates a high-resolution reverse banded pattern. The color images were captured by using the Photometrics cooled-CCD camera and BDS image analysis software (ONCOR Imaging, Gaithersburg, MD).

To determine whether a given individual carried a deletion, BAC probes for elastin (592D8) were hybridized simultaneously with one or both anchor BACs (1184P14 carrying D7S1870 and 1008H17 carrying FZD9) as well as BAC 239C10 recognizing the flanking duplications. More than 20 cells of high technical quality were evaluated for each individual and scored for presence, absence or intermediate signal from each probe on both chromosomes. Deletions were scored only when all 20 cells revealed absent signals.

PCR Analysis

All PCR primers were constructed as referenced or designed manually as shown in Table 6.4. PCR reactions carried out in a PTC-100TM (MJ Research). PCRs were performed in 25–1 reaction mixtures containing 0.5–1 M each primer and 0.5–1 U Taq in 10× PCR buffer and 25 μm each of dATP, dCTP, dTTP, dGTP (GIBCO BRL) with 1.5 mM MgCl$_2$. After initial denaturation (94°C for 2 min) and amplification for 30 cycles (94°C for 45 sec, 57°C for 60 sec, final extension 72°C for 10 min), products were resolved by gel electrophoresis on 1–3% ethidium bordide-stained NuSieve agarose gels.

Sequence Analysis

Sequencing the ends of BAC and PAC inserts directly: Sequencing primers that immediately flank the insert were designed from the SP6 and T7 RNA promoters and other sites within the vectors and were used to sequence BAC and PAC ends directly without subcloning. The primer sequences used were SP6, 5' gatttaggtgacactgtag 3', and T7, 5' taatacgactcactataggg 3'. The sequencing reactions were performed as described in the dsDNA Cycle Sequencing System (BRL) using 6 g of midiprep DNA for each SP6 and T7 reaction. Electrophoresis in 60-cm, six-percent denaturing polyacrylamide gels gave up to 350 bp of sequence at 55W.

The University of Oklahoma's Advanced Center for Genome Technology (ACGT) (http://www.genome.ou.edu/human.html, AC004166) produced the large-scale sequencing of BAC clone 239C10. DNA sequence for BAC 350L10 was obtained from the Washington University Genome sequencing Center, as a series of unlinked contigs available at http://genome.wustl.edu/pub/gscl/sequence/st.louis/human/preliminary/7. The sequence of ATRA (EST M28639) and BBG were obtained by using BLAST search in NCBI database with the end sequence of BAC 581A8 (http://www.ncbi.nih.gov).

Genes and Markers

Cosmids 129F5, 165B5, 82C2, 34B3, 128D2, 102F12, 135F3, 157F3, 237H1, 63F7, 82B11, 209C11, 47D1, 183E1, 160G4, and 15E11 were a generous gift from Lap-Chee Tsui (Osborne et al., 1997a, 1997b). The information for DNA markers of D7489M, D7489U, D7489L, STS1, STS2, STS3, D7S2714, and D7S1870 were obtained either from the literature or the MIT web site (Perez-Jurado et al., 1998; Osborne et al., 1996; Gilbert-Dussardier et al., 1995) (http://www-genome.wi.mit.edu/).

Table 6.4
Oligonucleotide PCR Table

Genes (bp)	Access number/ref	5′ Primer sequences	3′ Primer sequences	PCR fragment sizes
NCF1	U57835	GGCCCCGCTCTCTGCCCGCA	GCAAGGGCCGAGACGCTAGC	182
FKBP6 exon 9	Meng et al., 1998			
WSTF exon 20	Lu et al., 1998			
FZD9	U82169	TGTCAAGGTCAGGCAAGTGAG	CTCACCTCCTACCTTCCCCCTTCCCAGCCA	283
CPE-R	AB000712	CTTCAGCCCAGGGCCCCTGG	GCACAGGTCCCATTTATTGT	224
RVP1	BA000714	GCATGGACTGTGAAACCTCA	GCTAAAACGAGAGGCTTTA	170
STX1A	U87315	CCTGTTGTCTTGCGCTCTGGG	AGATACAAATGTTTATTCTAC	426
ELN exon 1	J02948	ATGGCGGGGTCTGACGGCGGCG	GGATCCGCTTCCCAGGGGTC	568
ELN exon 36	J02948	GGACTCACAGTGATGTGCACC	GGCGGCCATGACAGGTCAACC	828
LIMK1	U62292	CTTTGTGAAGCTGGAACACTGG	GTTCCTTGGACGTCACGGTTCC	1334
D7S613	G18333			
WSCR1	AF045555	AGCACAGAGACCACGACTCC	CTGCGTCAGCGCCGCAGTCA	160
H23535	G25613			
RFC2	AF045555	CCACTCGCCCACCCTCACGT	GCAGCTCACTAGGACATTCA	640
GTF2i-STS1, STS2, STS3	Perez-Jurado et al., 1998			
D7S1870	Z51768			
D7S489	z16646			
WI-9539	G11821			

Polymorphic Marker Analyses

Microsatellite analyses were conducted using D7S489(A,B,C), D7S1870, D7S653, D7S675, D7S849, D7S613, D7S2472, D7S2476. Primers were designed from publicly available sequences and labeled with one of the three following dyes: 6-Carboxyfluorescein, 6-carboxy-2′,4′,7′,4,7-hexachlorofluorescein, and N,N,N',N'-tetramethyl-6-carboxyrhodamine. A fourth dye 6-carboxy-X-rhodamine labeled the lambda phage size standard. Multiplex PCR reactions were carried out in solutions containing 10 mM Tris–HCl (pH 8.9), 50 mM KCl, 2.5 mM $MgCl_2$ 100 ng genomic DNA, 200 μM from each subject.

Notes

This work was performed at Share's Child Disability Center and supported by grants from the Department of Energy (DE-PG03-92ER-61402 and DE-FC03-96ER62294 to J. R. Korenberg) and the National Institute of Child Health and Human Development (HD33113, J. R. Korenberg). J. R. Korenberg holds the Geri and Richard Brawerman Chair in Molecular Genetics. The work was also supported partially by grant NHGIN HG00313 to B. Roe and grants from The Oak Tree Philanthropic Foundation, and Call Foundation to U. Bellugi, and the James S. McDonnell Foundation to U. Bellugi and J. R. Korenberg.

Illustrations and quotes not to be used without written permission from the author. Copyright Dr. Julie R. Korenberg.

References

Altschul, S. F., Madden, T., Schaffer, A., Zhang, J., Zhang, H., Miller, W., & Lipman, D. J. (1997). Gapped BLAST and PSI-BLAST: A new generation of protein database search programs. *Nucleic Acids Research, 25,* 3389–3402.

Bellugi, U., Klima, E. S., & Wang, P. P. (1996). Cognitive and neural development: Clues from genetically based syndromes. In D. Magnussen (Ed.), *The life-span development of individuals: Behavioral neurobiological, and psychosocial perspectives* (pp. 223–243). The Nobel Symposium. New York: Cambridge University Press.

Bellugi, U., Lichtenberger, L., Jones, W., Lai, Z., & St. George, M. (chap. 1). The neurocognitive profile of Williams Syndrome: A complex pattern of strengths and weaknesses.

Bellugi, U., Lichtenberger, L., Mills, D., Galaburda, A., & Korenberg, J. (1999a). Bridging cognition, brain and molecular genetics: Evidence from Williams syndrome. *Trends in Neurosciences, 22,* 197–207.

Bellugi, U., Losh, M., Reilly, J., & Anderson, D. (1998). Excessive use of linguistically encoded affect: Stories from young children with Williams syndrome (Technical Report CND-9801). University of California, San Diego, Center for Research in Language, Project in Cognitive and Neural Development.

Bellugi, U., Mills, D., Jernigan, T., Hickok, G., & Galaburda, A. (1999b). Linking cognition, brain structure and brain function in Williams syndrome. In H. Tager-Flusberg (Ed.), *Neurodevelopmental disorders: Contributions to a new framework from the cognitive neurosciences.* (pp. 111–136). Cambridge, MA: MIT Press.

Bellugi, U., & Wang, P. P. (1998). Williams syndrome: From cognition to brain to gene. In G. Edelman & B. H. Smith (Eds.), *Encyclopedia of Neuroscience,* CD-ROM version. New York: Elsevier.

Bellugi, U., Wang, P. P., & Jernigan, T. L. (1994). Williams syndrome: An unusual neuropsychological profile. In S. Broman & J. Grafman (Eds.), *Atypical cognitive deficits in developmental disorders: Implications for brain function* (pp. 23–56). Hillsdale, NJ: Erlbaum.

Botta, A., Novelli, G., Mari, A., Novelli, A., Sabani, M., Korenberg, J. R., Osborne, L., Digilio, M. C., Giannotti, A., & Dallapiccola, B. (1999). Detection of an atypical 7q11.23 deletion in Williams syndrome patients which does not include the STX1A and FZD9 genes. *Journal of Medical Genetics, 36,* 478–480.

Campbell, L., Potter, A., Ignatius, J., Dubowitz, V., & Davies, K. (1997). Genomic variation and gene conversion in spinal muscular atrophy: Implications for disease process and clinical phenotype. *American Journal of Human Genetics, 61,* 40–50.

Curran, M. E., Atkinson, D. L., Ewart, A. K., Morris, C. A., Leppert, M. F., & Keating, M. T. (1993). The elastin gene is disrupted by a translocation associated with supravalvular aortic stenosis. *Cell, 73,* 159–168.

Ewart, A. K., Jin, W., Atkinson, D. L., Morris, C. A., & Keating, M. T. (1994). Supravalvular aortic stenosis associated with a deletion disrupting the elastin gene. *Journal of Clinical Investigations, 83,* 1071–1077.

Ewart, A. K., Morris, C. A., Atkinson, D., Jin, W., Sternes, K., Spallone, P., Stock, A. D., Leppert, M., & Keating, M. T. (1993). Hemizygosity at the elastin locus in the developmental disorder, Williams syndrome. *Nature Genetics, 5,* 11–18.

Francke, U., Hsieh, C. L., Foellmer, B. E., Lomax, K. J., Malech, H. L., & Leto, T. L. (1990). Genes for two autosomal recessive forms of chronic granulomatous disease assigned to 1q25 (NCF2) and 7q11.23 (NCF1). *American Journal of Human Genetics, 47,* 483–492.

Francke, U., Yang-Feng, T. L., Brissenden, J. E., & Ulrich, A. (1986). Chromosomal mapping of genes involved in growth control. *Cold Spring Harbor Symposium on Quantitative Biology, 51,* 855–866.

Frangiskakis, J. M., Ewart, A. K., Morris, C. A., Mervis, C. B., Bertrand, J., Robinson, B. F., Klein, B. P., Ensing, G. J., Everett, L. A., Green, E. D., Proschel, C., Gutowski, N. J., Noble, M., Atkinson, D. L., Odelberg, S. J., & Keating, M. T. (1996). LIM-kinase hemizygosity implicated in impaired visuospatial constructive cognition. *Cell, 86,* 59–69.

Galaburda, A., & Bellugi, U. (chap. 5). Cellular and molecular cortical neuroanatomy in Williams Syndrome.

Galaburda, A. M., Wang, P. P., Bellugi, U., & Rossen, M. (1994). Cytoarchitectonic findings in a genetically based disorder: Williams syndrome. *NeuroReport, 5,* 758–787.

Gilbert-Dussardier, B., Bonneau, D., Gigaral, N., Le Merrer, M., Bonnet, D., Phillip, N., Serville, F., Verloes, A., Rossi, A., Ayme, S., Weissenbach, J., Mattei, M.-G., Lyonnet, S., & Munnich, A. (1995). A novel microsatellite DNA marker at locus D7S1870 detects hemizygosity in 75% of patients with Williams syndrome. *American Journal of Human Genetics, 56,* 542–543.

Gorlach, A., Lee, P. L., Roesler, J., Hopkins, P. J., Christensen, B., Green, E. D., Chanock, S. J., & Curnutte, J. T. (1997). A p47-phox pseudogene carries the most common mutation causing p47-phox-deficient chronic granulomatous disease. *Journal of Clinical Investigations, 100,* 1907–1918.

Hirayu, H., Seto, P., Magnusson, R. P., Filetti, S., & Rapoport, B. (1987). Molecular cloning and partial characterization of a new autoimmune thyroid disease-related antigen. *Journal of Clinical Endocrinology and Metabolism, 64,* 578–584.

Hoogenraad, C. C., Eussen, B. H., Langeveld, A., Haperen, R., Winterberg, S., Wouters, C. H., Grosveld, F., De Zeeuw, C. L., & Galjart, N. (1998). The murine CYLN2 gene: Genomic organization, chromosome localization and comparison to the human gene that is located within the 7q11.23 Williams syndrome critical region. *Genomics, 53,* 348–358.

Hubert, R. S., Mitchell, S., Chen, X.-N., Ekmekji, K., Gadomski, C., Sun, Z., Noya, D., Kim, U.-J., Chen, C., Shizuya, H., Simon, M., de Jong, P. J., & Korenberg, J. R. (1997). BAC and PAC contigs covering 3.5 Mb of the Down syndrome congenital heart disease region between D21S55 and MX1 on chromosome 21. *Genomics, 41,* 218–226.

Ishikawa, K., Nagase, T., Suyama, M., Tanaka, A., Kotani, H., Nomura, N., & Ohara, O. (1998). Prediction of the coding sequences of unidentified human genes: X. The complete sequences of 100 new cDNA clones from brain which can code for large proteins. *DNA Research, 176,* 169–176.

Jernigan, T. L., & Bellugi, U. (1994). Neuroanatomical distinctions between Williams and Down syndromes. In S. Broman and J. Grafman (Eds.), *Atypical cognitive deficits in developmental disorders: Implications in brain function* (pp. 57–66). Hillsdale, NJ: Erlbaum.

Jones, W., Bellugi, U., Lai, Z., Chiles, M., Reilly, J., Lincoln, A., & Adolphs, R. (chap. 2). Hypersociability: The social and affective phenotype of Williams Syndrome.

Korenberg, J. R., & Chen, X.-N. (1995). Localization of human CREBBP (CREB Binding Protein) to 16p13.3 by fluorescence in situ hybridization. *Cytogenetics and Cell Genetics, 71,* 56–57.

Korenberg, J. R., Chen, X.-N., Adams, M. D., & Venter, J. C. (1995). Towards a cDNA map of the human genome. *Genomics, 29,* 364–370.

Korenberg, J. R., Chen, X.-N., Lai, Z., Yimlamai, D., Bisighini, R., & Bellugi, U. (1997a). Williams syndrome. The search for genetic origins of cognition. *American Journal of Human Genetics, 61,* A103, 579.

Korenberg, J. R., Chen, X.-N., Mitchell, S., Sun, Z.-G., Hubert, R., Vataru, E. S., & Bellugi, U. (1996). The genomic organization of Williams syndrome. *American Journal of Medical Genetics Supplement, 59,* A306, 1776.

Korenberg, J. R., Chen, X.-N., Mitchell, S., Sun, Z.-G., Hubert, R., Vataru, E. S., & Bellugi, U. (1997b). The genomic organization of Williams syndrome. *International Behavioral Neuroscience Society Abstracts, 6,* 59, P2–52.

Korenberg, J. R., Chen, X.-N., Sun, Z., Shi, Z.-Y., Ma, S., Vataru, E., Yimlamai, D., Weissenbach, J. S., Shizuya, H., Simon, M. I., Gerety, S. S., Nguyen, H., Zemsteva, I. S., Hui, L., Silva, J., Wu, X., Birren, B., & Hudson, T. J. (1999a). Human genome anatomy: BACs integrating the genetic and cytogenetic maps for bridging genome and biomedicine. *Genome Research, 9(10),* 994–1001.

Korenberg, J. R., Lai, Z., & Bellugi, U. (1999b). In preparation.

Levitin, D. J., & Bellugi, U. (1998). Musical abilities in individuals with Williams syndrome. *Music Perception, 15,* 357–389.

Li, D. Y., Toland, A. E., Boak, B. B., Atkinson, D. L., Ensing, G. J., Morris, C. A., Keating, M. T. (1997). Elastin point mutations cause an obstructive vascular disease, supravalvular aortic stenosis. *Human Molecular Genetics, 6,* 1021–1028.

Lu, X., Meng, X., Morris, C. A., & Keating, M. T. (1998). A novel human gene, WSTF, is deleted in Williams syndrome. *Genomics, 54,* 241–249.

Lupski, J. R. (1998). Genomic disorders: Structural features of the genome can lead to DNA rearrangements and human disease traits. *Trends in Genetics, 10,* 417–422.

Meng, X., Lu, X., Li, Z., Green, E. D., Massa, H., Trask, B. J., Morris, C. A., & Keating, M. T. (1998a). Complete physical map of the common deletion region in Williams syndrome and identification and characterization of three novel genes. *Human Genetics, 103,* 590–599.

Meng, X., Lu, X., Morris, C. A., & Keating, M. T. (1998b). A novel human gene FKPB6 is deleted in Williams syndrome. *Genomics, 52,* 130–137.

Mills, D., Alvarez, T., St. George, M., Appelbaum, L., Bellugi, U., & Neville, H. J. (chap. 3). Neurophysiological markers of face processing in Williams Syndrome.

Morris, C. A., Leonard, C. O., & Dilates, C. (1988). Natural history of Williams syndrome: Physical characteristics. *Journal of Pediatrics, 113,* 318–325.

Morris, C. A., Loker, J., Ensing, G., & Stock, A. D. (1993). Supravalvular aortic stenosis cosegregates with familial 6; 7 translocation which disrupts the elastin gene. *American Journal of Medical Genetics, 46,* 737–744.

Neville, H. J., Mills, D., & Bellugi, U. (1994). Effects of altered auditory sensitivity and age of language acquisition on the development of language-relevant neural systems: Preliminary studies of Williams syndrome. In S. Broman & J. Grafman (Eds.), *Atypical cognitive deficits in developmental disorders: Implications for brain function* (pp. 67–83). Hillsdale, NJ: Erlbaum.

Nickerson, E., Greenberg, F., Keating, M. T., McCaskill, C., & Shaffer, L. G. (1995). Deletions of the elastin gene at 7q11.23 occur in approximately 90% of patients with Williams syndrome. *American Journal of Human Genetics, 56,* 1156–1161.

Nicolaides, N. C., Carter, K., Shell, B. K., Papadopoulos, N., Vogelstein, B., & Kinzler, K. W. (1995). Genomic organization of the human PMS2 gene family. *Genomics, 30,* 195–206.

Olson, T. M., Michels, V. V., Urban, Z., Csiszar, K., Christiano, A. M., Driscoll, D. J., Feldt, R. H., Boyd, C. D., Thibodeau, S. N. (1995). A 30 kb deletion within the elastin gene results in familial supravalvular aortic stenosis. *Human Molecular Genetics, 4,* 1677–1679.

Osborne, L. R., Herbrick, J. A., Greavette, T., Heng, H. H., Tsui, L.-C., & Scherer, S. W. (1997a). PMS2-related genes flank the rearrangement breakpoints associated with Williams syndrome and other diseases on human chromosome 7. *Genomics, 45,* 402–406.

Osborne, L. R., Martindale, D., Scherer, S. W., Shi, X. M., Huizenga, J., Heng, H. H. Q., Costa, T., Pober, B., Lew, L., Brinkman, J., Rommens, J., Koop, B., & Tsui, L.-C. (1996). Identification of genes from a 500-kb region at 7q11.23 that is commonly deleted in Williams syndrome patients. *Genomics, 36,* 328–336.

Osborne, L. R., Sodar, S., Shi, X.-M., Pober, B., Costa, T., Scherer, S. W., & Tsui, L.-C. (1997b). Hemizygous deletion of the syntaxin 1A gene in individuals with Williams syndrome. *American Journal of Human Genetics, 61,* 449–452.

Pankau, R., Partsch, D. J., Neblung, A., Gosch, A., & Wessel, A. (1994). Head circumference of children with Williams-Beuren Syndrome. *American Journal of Medical Genetics, 52,* 285–290.

Paperna, T., Peoples, R., Wang, Y. K., & Francke, U. (1998). Genes for the CPE receptor (CPETR$_1$) and the human homolog of RUP$_1$ (CPETR$_2$) are localized within the Williams-Beuren Syndrome deletion. *American Journal of Human Genetics, 54,* 453–459.

Peoples, R., Perez-Jurado, L., Wang, Y. K., Kaplan, P., & Francke, U. (1996). The gene for replication factor C subunit 2 (RFC2) is within the 7q11.23 Williams syndrome deletion. *American Journal of Human Genetics, 58,* 1370–1373.

Perez-Jurado, L. A., Wang, Y. K., Peoples, R., Coloma, A., Cruces, J., & Francke, U. (1998). A duplicated gene in the breakpoint regions of the 7q11.23 Williams-Beuren syndrome deletion encodes the initiator binding protein TFII-I and BAP-135, a phosphorylation target of BTK. *Human Molecular Genetics, 7,* 325–334.

Reilly, J. S., Klima, E. S., & Bellugi, U. (1990). Once more with feeling: Affect and language in atypical populations. *Development and Psychopathology, 2,* 367–391.

Reiss, A. L., Eliez, S., Schmitt, E. J., Strauss, E., Lai, Z., Jones, W. L., & Bellugi, U. (chap. 4). Neuroanatomy of Williams syndrome: A high-resolution MRI study.

Robinson, W. P., Waslynka, J., Bernasconi, F., Wang, M., Clark, S., Kotzot, D., & Schinzel, A. (1996). Delineation of 7q11.2 deletions associated with Williams-Beuren syndrome and mapping of a repetitive sequence to within and to either side of the common deletion. *Genomics, 34,* 17–23.

Tassabehji, M., Metcalfe, K., Donnai, D., Hurst, J., Reardon, W., Burch, M., & Read, A. P. (1997). Elastin: Genomic structure and point mutations in patients with supravalvular aortic stenosis. *Human Molecular Genetics, 7,* 1029–1036.

Tassabehji, M., Metcalfe, K., Karmiloff-Smith, A., Carette, M. J., Grant, J., Dennis, N., Reardon, W., Splitt, M., Read, A., & Donnai, D. (1999). Williams syndrome: Use of chromosomal microdeletions as a tool to dissect cognitive and physical phenotypes. *American Journal of Human Genetics, 64,* 118–125.

Wang, Y. K., Samos, C. H., Peoples, R., Perez-Jurado, L. A., Nusse, R., & Francke, U. (1997). A novel human homologue of the *Drosophila* frizzled wnt receptor gene binds wingless protein and is in the Williams syndrome deletion at 7q11.23. New Gene called F1/27/1993. *Human Molecular Genetics, 6,* 465–472.

Epilogue

Three Perspectives . . .

After completing this book, we were fortunate enough to have three leading scientists from the major fields of research brought together in this book (neuroscience, neuropsychology, and genetics) write down their reflections and opinions about what they read. They are David G. Amaral, Martha Denckla, and Christopher Wills.

A Neuroscience Perspective

Ursula Bellugi and colleagues have produced a volume that is not only a fascinating summary of their most recent findings on Williams Syndrome, but is also a blueprint for how all neurodevelopmental disorders could and should be investigated. This is a celebration of the integrated, multidisciplinary approach that will ultimately provide insight into the causes of the various cognitive abnormalities associated with the disorder and will also likely provide valuable new information on the genetic underpinnings of functions ranging from language to visuospatial processing to social behavior.

Williams Syndrome is a genetically based syndrome that is characterized by mild to moderate mental retardation. What is remarkable about Williams Syndrome is the "peaks and valleys" in the cognitive abilities of affected individuals. There is remarkably preserved and even elegant language function that contrasts with very poor mathematical ability. Perception of faces is normal, if not superior, and Williams Syndrome subjects are characteristically hypersocial and very trusting, often to the chagrin of their parents. On the other hand, visuo-spatial processing is impaired. These facts concerning the disorder have emerged from a comprehensive experimental neuropsychological assessment battery that Bellugi and colleagues have administered to their patient population. The same subjects have undergone electrophysiological, magnetic resonance imaging and molecular biological studies to search for any neurobiological alterations that might be associated with the changes in cognitive function. Electroencephalographic studies, for example, indicate altered responses to faces and abnormal cerebral specialization for language function. The structural imaging studies report a generally smaller brain with relative sparing of the cerebellum but volume reduction of parietal-occipital areas. Cortical gray matter appears to be preserved but there is a loss of cortical white matter. The overall distribution of cortical tissue may also be altered with a greater ratio of frontal to posterior cortex than in the normal controls. These changes provide a promissory note that more detailed investigations will highlight consistent structural alterations in the Williams Syndrome brain. Histological studies compliment these approaches, providing intriguing observations concerning dysmorphology of the cerebral cortex and volume changes in parietal/occipital areas as well as the amygdala. Finally, this volume ends with a description of the powerful molecular approaches pursued by Korenberg and colleagues to determine which of the genes deleted on chromosome 7 may be associated with the various cognitive dysfunctions and biological alterations that have been found to characterize Williams Syndrome.

Faced with a biologically and cognitively complex neurodevelopmental syndrome, Bellugi and colleagues have created a multidisciplinary scientific team and have explicitly designed research strategies that take the collaboration from genes to neural systems to higher cognitive function, with reaches in the future to management, treatment, and perhaps even prevention. While the journey is not yet over, I believe that neuroscientists, cognitive scientists, molecular biologists, physicians, therapists, and parents alike will be fascinated by the sights along the way.

David G. Amaral, Ph.D.
Professor of Psychiatry and Neuroscience
University of California, Davis
Davis, California

A Neuropsychology Perspective

This book exemplifies a relatively recent development in cognitive neuroscience—the attempt to move from gene to brain to observable manifestations of cognition. Within this new enterprise, the research program led by Ursula Bellugi and her multidisciplinary group of colleagues represents the most sophisticated and successful effort to date. Utilizing the most advanced molecular biology, this research group fills in almost every available scientific "blank" on the pathophysiology "form" that connects to what in Williams syndrome is strikingly spared (language, sociability) and impaired (visuospatial ability).

Starting with the inspired design in which an IQ-matched contrast group (Down Syndrome) proved to have a markedly different profile from that of Williams Syndrome, Bellugi et al. chipped away at the thought-restricting monolith of "mental retardation." The effective use of qualitative characteristics, more telling than level of performance, as discriminative data stands as another of the Bellugi group's pioneering contributions to neurogenetic research.

Now, this series of chapters have carried the story of Williams Syndrome further, with the addition of several novel and important approaches. The structural neuroimaging is "next generation" from that which has previously been employed with Williams Syndrome. Structure is microscopically explored by Galaburda, the acknowledged national expert on developmental neuropathology. Sure enough, the Mills et al. electrophysiological chapter confirms the suspicion that language processing and social orientation are mediated by anomalous neural circuits in Williams Syndrome. The anatomical and physiological evidence converge nicely. The longitudinal aspect of the group's research is a vital testimony to the principle of developmental cognitive neuroscience; that how a profile unfolds is as important a clue to pathophysiology as is the "final status" profile.

Another remarkable contribution of the first three chapters (Bellugi et al., Jones et al., Mills et al.) taken together is that they are chipping away at yet another outdated "monolith," the Nonverbal Learning Disabilities. This "chipping" consists of the separation of social from spatial cognition, heretofore lumped together. The "monolith" of Nonverbal Learning Disabilities, so effectively called into question by the Bellugi group's work on Williams Syndrome, has in other hands become a kind of rationale for stagnation as regards measures of social orientation (sociability) and social competence. It is always dangerous to assume that we know what we do not know; the Williams syndrome profile is a warning against such complacency.

Finally, the example of Williams Syndrome as a model of a chromosomal deletion leading to a visuospatial deficit has sparked inquiries into variation among the spatially-inept in a college freshman cohort for the chromosome band 7q11.23. Another group seeks to scrutinize parental (maternal vs. paternal) source of the X chromosome in Turner Syndrome as a source of variation in spatial aptitude. Such are the sparks given off by the research represented in this book, an inspiration for all who labor to understand behavioral phenotypes.

Martha Denckla
Professor of Neurology, Pediatrics, and Psychiatry
John Hopkins University School of Medicine
Baltimore, Maryland

An Evolutionary Perspective

The first thing that should be pointed out is that the children and adults with Williams, and their families, by giving so unstintingly of their time, have provided science and medicine with an unprecedented opportunity to learn important information about the nature of language and the way the brain works. They should be very proud of the results that are presented in this volume, which are sure to have important consequences for our understanding of Williams and similar syndromes.

What is, I think, really exciting about these studies is that they enable us to begin to examine these mysterious developmental pathways. Williams is a particularly clear-cut case of genetic damage that affects only parts of the brain. There are many other deletions with dramatic consequences on brain function that have been found scattered along our chromosomes and that lead to a wide variety of retardation syndromes—Angelman,

Langer-Giedon, Prader-Willi, and so on. Close examination of the genetics of these other deletions is likely to lead to the ability to dissect brain function in other ways.

The genetic studies in this volume are superbly complemented by the studies of brain function (Reiss et al.) and brain structure (Galaburda and Bellugi). The importance of the cerebellum in cognitive function is of particular evolutionary interest, because it demonstrates that many changes at every level have happened to our brains in the course of evolution. The simplistic notion that all our increased intellectual capacity is the result of an increase in the size of the cortex has been laid to rest!

Another point raised by these studies is a more directly evolutionary one. It appears that this region of chromosome 7 is prone to both deletions and duplications, in part because it is flanked by repeat regions. The situation is extremely complex, including nested deletions that involve part of the WMS region and the conversion of some of the duplicated genes into pseudogenes. Further, massive rearrangements of the chromosome and of the Williams region have occurred in the course of primate evolution. Perhaps the most dramatic changes have been a substantial chromosomal inversion and a duplication of part of the Williams region that have taken place in the lineage that leads to the chimpanzees and ourselves.

What remains to be seen is whether all these rearrangements are simply part of the continuing rearrangement of the genome that accompanies speciation in any group of organisms, or whether this region might be involved in the very rapid evolution of human (and chimpanzee) cognitive function. I am intrigued that a "core" segment of the WMS region, including the elastin gene, has been preserved as a single functional copy throughout this complex process, while flanking regions have become duplicated. This suggests that nonrandom forces have been at work and indicates that this region is a very important one.

Genetic damage must be severe to produce a permanent deficit, and a surprisingly small number of genetic conditions account for the majority of cases of gene-caused mental retardation. This means that the developmental pathways leading to the brain must be remarkably redundant. If a deficit in any one of the tens of thousands of genes that are involved in brain development and function were to result in severe damage, none of us would escape unscathed. The study of Williams will lead us to a fuller understanding of this redundancy and to a deeper understanding of how we can take full advantage of this astonishing evolutionary gift.

Christopher Wills
Professor of Biology
University of California, San Diego
La Jolla, California

Where do we go from here . . .

Thus, our goal to build bridges across disciplines, linking higher cognitive functions, their underlying neurobiological bases, and their molecular genetic underpinnings, is finally visible on the horizon. We have entered the era in which the compelling vision of understanding the effects of specific genes on human development, cognition, and behavior may in principle be realized. This will of course be a complex process requiring unprecedented and intensive multidisciplinary effort. Techniques for identifying gene function and interaction will be expanded and improved. Innovative methods for visualization and measurement of micro- and macro-anatomy of the brain will be utilized. Neurocognitive and behavioral measures with greater correspondence to biological constructs will be developed. It is likely that the next decade will oversee mapping of specific neurocognitive functions and underlying neural systems to particular genes within critical deletion regions. We look forward to this exciting time and contribution.

Editors and Authors

Editor names, positions, and affiliations

Ursula Bellugi Dr. Bellugi is a Professor at The Salk Institute for Biological Studies. She is also Director of the Laboratory for Cognitive Neuroscience at the Salk Institute. Her doctorate is from Harvard University in Cognitive Psychology and Education. Her laboratory focuses on linking cognition, brain, and gene in individuals with Williams Syndrome, as well as on studies of the neurobiology of sign language and other cognitive processes in the brain. Her research has received a Distinguished Scientific Contribution Award and the Prize in Neuronal Plasticity from the IPSEN Foundation. She has written more than 200 papers and authored several books including *The Signs of Language, Spatial Cognition: Brain Basis and Development,* and *What the Hands Reveal About the Brain.*

Marie St. George, Ph.D. Dr. St. George is a Research Scientist at the University of California, San Diego, with special focus on language comprehension using brain imaging techniques including event-related brain potentials and functional magnetic resonance imaging. Her Ph.D. is in Cognitive Psychology from the University of Delaware, and she is the author of several papers on Williams Syndrome.

Primary Author Biographies

Ursula Bellugi, Ed.D. Chapter 1 (see above)

Wendy Jones, Ph.D. Chapter 2 Dr. Jones has a Ph.D. from the Joint Doctoral Program in Clinical Psychology at San Diego State University and the University of California, San Diego, and is a research scientist in the Laboratory for Cognitive Neuroscience at The Salk Institute for Biological Studies. She has been involved in clinical and research studies for many years, and has published papers on language, affect, and the brain in Williams Syndrome.

Debra Mills, Ph.D. Chapter 3 Dr. Mills is a Research Scientist at the Center for Research in Language, University of California, San Diego, and an Associate Professor of Psychology at Emory University. She has a Ph.D. from UCSD in Psychology and a previous position at the Salk Institute for Biological Studies in the Laboratory for Neuropsychology. Dr. Mills specializes in the neurophysiological underpinnings of human cognition, using event-related potentials (ERPs) to examine brain function. Her laboratory focuses on the development of cerebral specializations for language, nonlanguage cognitive functions, and sensory processing in normal and atypical infants, children, and adults.

Allan L. Reiss, M.D. Chapter 4 Dr. Reiss is Director of the Division of Child and Adolescent Psychiatry and Child Development, and the Howard C. Robbins Professor in Psychiatry and Behavioral Sciences at Stanford University School of Medicine. He also is Director of the Stanford Psychiatry Neuroimaging Laboratory and the Behavioral Neurogenetics Research Program. He is a graduate of Swarthmore College and George Washington University School of Medicine. Dr. Reiss has worked extensively, in both research and clinical settings, with individuals affected by developmental, genetic, and neuropsychiatric disorders including Williams Syndrome. His areas of expertise include describing the behavioral and cognitive profiles of individuals with these disorders, the use of structural and functional brain imaging techniques to uncover and elucidate neural mechanisms, and linking genetic, neurobiological, and neurobehavioral data to more fully understand the neurodevelopmental pathways leading to cognitive and behavioral disability in these conditions.

Albert M. Galaburda, M.D. Chapter 5 Dr. Galaburda is the Emily Fischer Landau Professor of Neurology and Neuroscience at Harvard Medical School. He is also the Chief of the Division of Behavioral Neurology, which includes the Dyslexia Neuroanatomical Research Laboratory at Beth Israel Deaconess Medical Center in Boston, Massachusetts. Dr. Galaburda received his M.D. from Boston University following internships under the direction of Norman Geschwind. His research areas include the neurobiological foundations of cerebral dominance, developmental dyslexia and related learning disorders, experimental developmental neuropathology, cerebral architectonics and connectivity, genetics of behavioral disorders, and the organization of knowledge in the central nervous system. Dr. Galaburda has been awarded the Fellow of the Royal Society of Medicine, Scientist of the Year, ACLD, Pattison Prize in Neuroscience. He is author of more than 150 journal articles, book chapters, and several books including *Cerebral Lateralization, Cerebral Dominance; From Reading to Neurons; Neurobiology of Cognition;* and *The Extraordinary Brain, Normal and Abnormal Development of the Cortex.*

Julie R. Korenberg, Ph.D., M.D. Chapter 6 Dr. Korenberg is Vice Chair of Pediatrics for Research, and the Brawerman Chair in Molecular Genetics at Cedars-Sinai Medical Center. She is also a Professor of Pediatrics and Human Genetics at the University of California at Los Angeles. Dr. Korenberg earned a Ph.D. from the University of Wisconsin, and an M.D. from the University of Miami. She is a world-renowned geneticist and scientist who recently "pieced together the genome jigsaw" by developing a comprehensive color-coded map to the human genome, which is featured in *Genome Research, Nature,* and *Science.* She has over 120 publications and has authored chapters for several encyclopedias and medical books, holds memberships in several professional organizations including the American Society of Human Genetics, and was recently honored by Hadassah as Woman of the Year for her pioneering research.

Index